Finding Rainbows in Storm Clouds

25 Life Lessons I Learned from a Brain Tumor

Erin Pizzo

ISBN: 069265626X
ISBN 13: 978-0692656266

Finding Rainbows in Storm Clouds

Dedication 5

Medical Disclaimer 6

Introduction 7

Phoenix Burning 10

Phoenix Rising 17

1. Vibration is Your Signature Scent 33

2. The Body Is a Biofeedback System 39

3. I Remembered God 44

4. Sometimes Rebooting Is the Easiest Answer 47

5. Don't Wait for Perfect Timing 51

6. Solitude Unleashes Your Inner Guru 54

7. Your Life Is Like a Movie 58

8. I am Not Fearless, but I Know How to Use My Fear 60

9. We Reap What We Sow 63

10. Don't Attach to Pain 66

11. I Am the Proverbial Onion 68

12. Play like Your Life Depends on It 70

13. Messages from the Ethers 72

14. Focus on What You Want, Not on What You Don't 78

15. Stop Proving Your Worth 83

16. Love the Ordinary 86

17. Soften, Don't Harden to Life 90

18. The Pursuit of Happiness Was Making Me Unhappy 92

19. Breaking Out of My Ego's Box of Fear 95

20. Seek Information, Not Affirmation 98

21. Parenting: The Fast Track to Spiritual Enlightenment 103

22. Bless It All 109

23. Make Love, Not War 112

24. Choice Chaos 114

25. A Tumor Is Like a Pearl..116

Afterword...118

Acknowledgments...119

Dedication

This book is dedicated to my amazing children, Aidan and Kyra. Thank you for choosing me to travel on your life journeys with you. It is my greatest honor!

Medical Disclaimer

The information in this book is for informational purposes only. It is not intended to be a substitute for professional medical advice or treatment. Always seek the advice of a qualified health-care provider with any questions you may have regarding a health condition.

Introduction

Before 2009 my life mantra was 'I am one of those people for whom nothing great and nothing terrible would ever happen'. For the record, I was wrong on both counts.

What if a brain tumor was the perfect vehicle to drive a radical shift in my consciousness? Because that is what it did! Was it the easiest way? No, but I would have ignored easier ways just like most other people. I have found that the vast majority of us won't change without our environment becoming incredibly hostile to the status quo. The brain tumor was the vehicle I was given to transform my life. I consider it a great blessing. Was it easy when it began? No. Is it an easy journey every day? Definitely not, but it has been a mind-blowing and amazing ride that finally woke me from my slumber, that finally kicked me in the ass enough to decide that I couldn't waste any more time.

The idea of inspiring others with my life journey would have been laughable prior to the brain tumor diagnosis. I was *terrified* of life. I lived as small a life as possible because that was the way I perceived I was safest. I was negative, afraid, and angry. The picture of inspiration, right?

Growth really only happens when we are uncomfortable. Many of us are living lives much smaller than we are meant to. I don't mean we all need to strive to be like Oprah. When I say smaller, I mean fitting in or hiding our real selves. Challenges aren't punishments; they are wake-up calls, they are serious soul growth pushing us to get in touch and then start radiating out our authentic selves, the people we are when we aren't trying to impress anyone. My experience is that those who face big challenges are amazing bad asses who just don't realize how awesome they are. It's painful for sure, but the people who have made great strides for humanity in history faced enormous challenges. The most inspiring people in your life are also probably those who have walked through fire.

Being diagnosed with a brain tumor was a fantastic way to disconnect from daily life stress. It gave me an entirely new perspective and forced me to reevaluate my priorities. It's easy to get caught up in the minutia of day to day life. It's easy to believe that pursuing a career, transporting children from activity to activity, performing well in school and extracurricular activities, paying bills, and buying nice homes, cars, and clothing is all there is, but then something comes along that knocks the perspective right into you. I used to be consumed by those details just like everybody else. Now I live with a balance of helping my children to be fulfilled and healthy, embracing day-to-day tasks, while nurturing my body and my soul. I can't hate the challenging days because of the way the challenges force me open and strip away any semblance of security I mistakenly believed I had. Security is both the absolute truth and an illusion to me now. It is truth because no matter what happens, we are a part of the matrix of the universe, even when we leave our physical bodies. That whole death thing? It's a terrible illusion. Sure, those who have passed on no longer physically reside here, but they are most definitely still present. I find that to be profoundly comforting. Everything is always in divine order. Security is an illusion simultaneously because we believe we can control our life circumstances. God (Source, universe or whatever name you subscribe to) will do what is best for each of us even when it looks like God is shredding our life to pieces.

We collectively do a pretty lame job of nurturing our souls. Often it's relegated to an hour on the weekend. The soul is treated like an afterthought in modern society, but without the soul, life is a series of random occurrences strung together without meaning. The soul is our guiding light.

This book is very much about unlearning, about peeling back the layers of crud our lives are coated with, so that we can remember our amazing power as sparks of God playing the game of life. When I wake up in the morning, I ask: "What would make my soul joyful today?" Some days I don't get it right. Some days I get stuck in the minutia; I'm human. More often than not, the answer is writing and helping others to find balance, peace and acceptance. When I help others, when I inspire someone to accept who she really is, to dive into the deep end, to trust, and to believe in herself, I feel radiant. Life truly is about the journey every day, the moments that happen now and not about the destination.

My sincere hope is that this book helps you to tap into the river of wisdom running within you, to clear out your clutter, and to remember that you are far more powerful than you probably ever allowed yourself to believe.

Love,

Erin

Phoenix Burning

I am like a phoenix. I rise from the ashes.

Bess Myerson

I have learned a lot from my challenge about living an authentic, inspired life, but first I need to explain the purification by fire that I had to go through before I could become like a phoenix rising from the ashes. Is suffering necessary for growth? It depends on how stubborn and stuck in your ways you are. I needed to suffer. I would never have had the courage to change without it.

These first two chapters describe my former self and the events that burned her to the ground. I do not like to dredge up the past, I used to, three years ago even I would have relished in sharing my burden with you, knowing that I would receive your sympathy, but you cannot heal anything with the same consciousness that created it. I was a complainer. I was a victim. If I want to change my life, I have to change the way I talk, think and feel about my life. With that said, you won't understand my transformation unless I share the darkness first. I can look at these events with love and humor now, as if "did this all truly fucking happen?" My lighter perspective is the only reason I am able to share it. Please don't see me as a victim. I am not. Do I wish sometimes that the tumor hadn't manifested? Yes I do, but, and it's a big but, my life was on the wrong trajectory. I have been honored and blessed with so many gifts as a direct result of this experience. I have found a peace that I never had before. I have found a love for myself and humanity that I never had before. I have been stunned by the awesome power of the unseen universe and the connection to the Divine that I now have. It is truly a great honor. Please don't get my story mixed up with my message. My message is that everything can be an opportunity or an obstacle. It all depends on how you choose to look at it. Cue the dramatic music...

Prior to 2009, I was living a very ordinary middle-class suburban American lifestyle. I am married to a great guy named Mike. We have two bright and funny kids, Aidan and Kyra. My husband commuted an hour each way to Boston every day, and I stayed home with our kids. These are *first world* problems I realize, but that's something I've learned. Your surroundings can easily mask low self-esteem and self-loathing. The trust fund baby can be more miserable than the guy working a 12 hour job. I recognize the privilege of being a stay-at-home mom and understand that some women would do anything to be able to do what I was doing, but it required a great deal of financial sacrifice and personal patience. While I adore my kids, the early years of babies, toddlers, and preschoolers were draining for me. Add to that being surrounded by mothers—many of whom were former teachers with a special talent for the wee ones and who seemed to always have their shit together—and you can imagine how my self-esteem plummeted. I admit these seem like trivial problems, but our perception is what creates our reality, and mine was that I wasn't good enough. I felt inadequate. I felt tremendous guilt that my children deserved a better mother. I lived in a slow downward spiral of self-pity and self-loathing. I didn't see options; I saw limitations. This was my self-constructed prison.

At 5:00 p.m. each day after not using any of my many years of education, I couldn't wait to reward myself with a tall white wine spritzer. I realize that hardly puts me in the camp of alcoholic, but I honestly believe that if you develop that much of an emotional need for something, it is, in fact, a problem. I was also addicted to *The West Wing* reruns on Bravo, quietly imagining myself as C. J. Cregg, kick-ass press secretary for President Bartlett.

The self-loathing I harbored was quite literally eating me alive. It's something I had felt since earliest childhood. I was the third of three daughters. My two older sisters were talented, organized, and competitive. I wasn't particularly any of those traits, at least in the way outsiders would notice. As you would expect after two daughters, it was also hoped that I was a boy. My parents loved me dearly, and my family always treated me lovingly. Any self-loathing I harbored was my own creation.

11

We expect children with difficult backgrounds to be messed up, but even children from idyllic settings can have emotional wounds that outsiders would never expect. I'm fairly certain there are a lot of people like me out there. I personally believe a lot of our illnesses are indications of self-loathing and fear on a deep subconscious level. If you are one of these people, please know that your past experiences, even and especially the painful ones, are powerful vehicles to bring you to where you are meant to be—to a life that fulfills you—if you are willing to be honest about how those experiences shaped you. You can choose to make your pain and self-loathing invisible to others too with the right mask, which is what I did. Eventually something will give. In my case, God was about to step in and rip off my mask.

I believe that God creates challenges to bring us closer to our true selves. I believe there is meaning to every experience. I believe the things we can't explain are beyond our limited ability to see the big picture, but that doesn't mean there isn't a purpose for them. I believe there is a soul component to our experiences, even those of babies and children. Does that make it one iota easier for the parents whose child has just died? No, but maybe it helps just a bit to believe that there is a plan, that their agony was not about the amusement of the gods. Maybe it helps just a bit to know that their child will always be with them. I don't see challenges as any form of punishment. Challenges provide serious soul growth. I would not have grown if my feet weren't held to the flames. Purification requires intense flames. I had a lot of purifying to do in both mind and body, so things were about to get unbearably hot in my life.

In 2009, my dear father, my Steady Eddie and very much a rock in my life, was diagnosed with stage IV lung cancer at the age of sixty-four. To see him, you would never know anything was wrong. He had no symptoms. The cancer was discovered on a routine chest x-ray. The night of his diagnosis is still the only night of my life where I could not sleep at all. Instead, I paced all night in my in-laws' house in Vermont where we were visiting for the Fourth of July weekend.

Stress has a profound effect on the human body. I don't say that intellectually. I *know* that. I have lived that. It is a truth I wish for everyone to understand and appreciate. There are times in your life that feel unbearable with stress, and fear and pain. There isn't a damn thing you can do to avoid it. It's incredibly important to find an outlet to release it, writing in a journal or cardio come to mind, rather than walking around with it in your body like a ticking time bomb. The day I learned of my father's diagnosis my body shook. In the next year, I went from sobbing to numbness to researching everything I could find about lung cancer, prognoses, possible new treatments, and my risk of cancer now that I was *genetically predisposed*. It was an endless loop. It became my obsession. Looking back, I am pretty sure I cried almost every day of my father's illness.

After six weeks of testing and second opinions, my father began a grueling regimen of chemotherapy. From the start, although I knew nothing about holistic cancer cures, I was against chemotherapy for him. I knew what stage IV meant, and I simply didn't see the point. He was a perfectly fine functioning human. Why destroy what time he had left? One must ask, if the treatment is worse than the disease AND won't heal you, why do it? Alas my father was a rule follower. If doctors recommended chemotherapy, he was going to do it.

Whether it is ethical to encourage a stage IV patient to use a very taxing treatment that may only marginally extend his life (six to nine months without treatment and twelve months with treatment) while destroying his quality of life, I will leave for you to decide, but in my mind, for him, it wasn't worth it. After just three weeks of chemotherapy, my father was a shell of himself. It was staggering to witness and further fueled my own body's stressful slide downward.

This was one of the observations I felt most conflicted about sharing. I know that most people feel intense pressure to use chemotherapy and I know many people who have healed after using it. Obviously, you can tell I believe there are other methods of healing that are preferable, but what you believe about something gives it power. If you decide to do chemotherapy, thank it, honor it and treat it like a magical healing elixir from God.

Sometimes people come to me and want me to help them choose a healing path. I share resources, but I will not tell people what to do. It is not *my* decision to make and I would never want someone to start chemotherapy with a toxic attitude toward it even though I would want them to know there are other routes. The unfair part from my perspective is that medical oncology does not share those other routes with their patients to offer choices even though they exist and work. I don't think it's the doctors, but the medical establishment which is heavily influenced by pharmaceutical companies, that are not inclined, nor qualified to counsel patients on healing nutrition nor any other natural support. Not only have they not studied it, but there is also no profit in it. I am actually not anti-conventional medicine. I am intrigued by the growth in immunotherapy. Cancer is big business. Pharmaceutical companies are publicly-traded and responsible to shareholders before patients. There will not be a pharmaceutical 'cure' unless they can find a way to profit from it.

Six weeks into the eight-week course of chemotherapy, I attended my husband's sister's wedding in Vermont. My parents were supposed to attend, but only my mother could make it. My father was far too weak. The day after the wedding, I drove to Albany, New York, to see him. He looked like death. He was too sick to walk, eat, or even sit up. He said to me, "Erin, I'm dying." That, right there, broke my heart into a million pieces. I tried to tell him that it was the effects of chemotherapy, not the cancer, that was making him feel like that, but the man was as stubborn as a mule. It was, in fact, the chemotherapy and not the cancer, because only two weeks later, he was taken off the regimen because it failed to stop the cancer from growing. Once he transitioned to the second-line chemotherapy regimen—a far gentler version—he recovered much of his vigor.

My father had his ups and downs for several months after that. By May 2010, it became clear that his health was failing. The cancer spread to his brain, and he began whole head radiation. The steroids altered his personality dramatically. My cautious father went wild with purchases and also became angry. It was the steroids. They gave him energy, but also really messed with his decision making. I also witnessed him eating more sugar than I thought humanly possible.

Around this time, I asked my hairdresser to lighten my hair. That might sound rather *out of the blue*, but for most of my life, my father had known me as a blonde. I needed his last images of me to be as he had always known me. While washing my hair, my hairdresser noticed an egg-size bump on my skull. It didn't hurt, but I was surprised I had never noticed it before. By this time, I was as jumpy as a dog around fireworks. My doctor took pity on me, knowing the state of my father's health, and scheduled me for an MRI out of sympathy more than anything else.

I remember that the MRI was located in the basement of a medical building and that I had never been so claustrophobic in my life. I asked the technicians to talk to me during the scan, but they didn't. They also didn't look me in the eye afterward. I should have read the signals. When I got my results the next day, a five-centimeter white matter lesion, I was numb. It wasn't known yet whether it was brain cancer or tumefactive multiple sclerosis. The truth is, on some level I expected it. It almost seemed inevitable. I was on a trajectory with doom.

I had been hiding my true self. I had been parading around as a victim. God was lighting a fire under me because I refused to heed the subtler guidance that I was receiving through my feelings. When we fail to listen to the quieter messages, they get louder and more difficult to ignore until you have no choice but to change. God was asking and wanting more from me than I had been giving to life. It is reminiscent of the stories of captains burning their ships upon arriving on new shores so that their crew had no choice but to make life work or perish. Many people we admire publicly went through very difficult events in their lives that sharpened their resolve. People like Oprah Winfrey, Thomas Edison, Jim Carrey, and even Franklin Delano Roosevelt experienced personal horrors, significant challenges, or professional failures time and again.

Not everybody heeds the call to purify. Some choose to go deeper into the victim mentality and give more power away. But if you can embrace the call, what you will learn and the ways in which you will grow will be like jumping from remedial math to calculus. It's not an easy or well laid out process. You make it up as you go along. It is messy. It is painful. It is lonely because most people in your life want to continue to follow the beaten path. Many people think they know what's best for you and try to steer you back onto the familiar path. They mean well, but they add far more pressure and pain to an already intensely difficult situation. They do it out of love for you and fear of the unknown. With time, they either get behind you or you distance yourself from them. Forging your own trail is a pioneering business, and pioneers spend a lot of time alone. It is an intense process of releasing the shackles that YOU held yourself in. At some point you finally realize that the only key you need is to be yourself...*authentically*.

When we are living authentically and purposefully, the gifts we came here to share spill out of us with very little effort. I am no guru. I am not better than anyone else, but rather than throw myself a pity party, I chose to see an opportunity instead of an obstacle. I want to help you do the same.

<u>Phoenix Rising</u>

I began the battery of tests and appointments that all new diagnoses bring. Now, not only was I shuttling back and forth from the Boston area to Albany, New York, to be with my father, but I was juggling appointments and extremely raw nerves. Between my first and second neurology appointments I lost eight pounds. Some people eat under extreme stress, I lose my appetite completely. I lost so much weight that the neurologist commented on it.

I shared my health news with my sisters, friends, and my husband's parents, but kept it from my mother who had enough to worry about. I also, naturally, didn't burden my father with this news. Three days after my bombshell, my father fell and was admitted to the St. Peter's Hospital hospice wing, the most compassionate and lovely place to transition, where they even allowed my father's beloved golden retriever to visit. *This was one year to the day of his diagnosis.*

The timing is no coincidence in my opinion—it's textbook nocebo effect. Maybe you've heard of the placebo effect where a patient will get better with a sugar pill that he or she believes is medicine? Not only is this remarkably common, but someone I know in the pharmaceutical sales world told me that often the placebo is *just as effective* as the approved drug. The nocebo effect refers to when someone is given bad news, such as a grim prognosis, and responds on cue. My father's oncologist had given him one year to live with treatment and six to nine months without. My father did the treatments and, like the good patient he was, passed when he was told he would. The power of suggestion is vast. Some might say that just means the doctors knew what they were talking about. I'm not so sure about that. Prognoses are tricky business. Prognoses do not account for the people who walk away from the conventional medical complex and simply don't check in again. The will to live, even among those who do conventional treatments, has been seen to affect the outcome. Patients often want to know the hard facts, and yet for as much as they want them, hard facts simply do not account for individual will. A

17

prognosis thus becomes an albatross around the patient's neck, another obstacle to healing.

I left for Albany, New York, directly from an MRI when my sister called to tell me that my father had fallen. The level of despair that I felt is difficult to describe. It honestly felt like life could never be good again. For the next few days, I practically lived at the hospital. I remember crying in the family common room one day. One of the grief counselors came over to console me. Grief counselors are a special breed of hero in my book. I told him everything. It helped me so much to release it all, as I had been feeling like an island, alone and terrified. I couldn't unload my burden on my sisters who were managing their own grief. I also had no friends nearby. I didn't even have my husband there to support me as we thought it was best for him to stay with the kids in Massachusetts since we had no way of knowing how long my father might hang on.

On July 5, 2010, I said goodbye to my father to head back to Boston for more tests. I remember questioning whether I should stay or go, but feeling like I needed to get some answers. To be perfectly honest, I was hoping someone would tell me "oops, we were wrong", but that didn't happen. My father had been spending most of his time removed from his body. I know that sounds *out there*, but it is the truth. If you have been with loved ones at the end of their lives, you are probably familiar with the way they slip in and out of consciousness. For the three days I was with him at the hospital, he was mostly unconscious. I now understand more that he was in between planes of consciousness. I only saw him coherent three times in those days. The first was when his dear friend and family priest came to visit. My father was able to communicate, albeit in a fractured way. The second was when my baby nephew came to see him. The third was when I said goodbye to him.

Having read the near-death account of Anita Moorjani,[1] I now believe that my father was completely aware of my health issue at the time. As we transition, we move out of our bodies and can be many places at once. I have no doubt that he heard my conversations with the grief counselor in the common room, with family friends who came to say goodbye…all of it. My father was no longer confined to his body.

When it was time to say goodbye, I was startled that he rolled over to me on his right side and reached out to hug me. He also tried to talk, but all that came out was a *huff*. I told him that it was okay to go if it was his time, but that I would be back in two days if he wanted to hang on. I also told him how blessed I felt that he had been my father.

As I left the hospital alone that day, nowhere near my father's room, a young man ran up behind me and said, "Excuse me, miss? God asked me to tell you God bless you." I was speechless, which, as someone who loves to write and speak, was frustrating. I sure do wish I'd thought to ask him some questions, but instead I said "thank you", and that was it. I heard him go back to his friends and say, "I think she thinks I'm nuts". I didn't think that, but I wondered what my divine message meant. Did it mean my father would miraculously recover? Did it mean the doctors were wrong about me? Or did it mean all the shit was truly hitting the fan, but that God wanted me to know that He was with me. I was perplexed, yet comforted.

The next day, I had the most painful experience of my life, a poorly executed spinal tap in the neurologist's office. I asked for pain management before we started, but was told it wouldn't be necessary. When he stuck the needle in, I screamed bloody murder. I have been through labor and epidurals. That was child's play compared to this. He made a mistake that I won't share, but I was very traumatized and, again, felt like an island with no support.

The day after the spinal tap, I headed back to Albany on July 7, 2010, directly from an MRI. I was alone in the car. I called my sister to tell her when to expect me and she told me my father was unconscious, but alive. Just after I hung up, I experienced the most significant moment of my life. I felt a wave of energy rush through me from left to right. I went from a state of deep despair to euphoria. I had no idea what was going on. I turned on the radio and started singing along to Top 40 hits. I even remember asking myself, *Why are you so happy? You are going to your father's deathbed and you likely have a brain tumor!*

Nevertheless, nothing could shake my mood. I practically skipped into the hospital and up to my father's room. Just outside his door, I saw my sister's face, however, and knew that my father had passed. I found out that he passed forty-five minutes earlier, at the time my euphoria began, and I *knew*. I knew that somehow, my father had shared his passing with me. It was one of the most precious moments of my life, up there with the births of my children. In that moment I *Knew* (with a capital *K*) that death is not real and that our soul goes on. Game changer…

I spent some time alone in my father's room. As odd as this might sound, I lay down on the bed with him and hugged him. It is such a strange sensation to lie with someone perfectly still, without the movement of breath. I turned on his iPod and just lay there wishing so much that this was all a bad dream. I stayed at the hospital with my sister Sue to await the funeral home staff, while my mother and my sister Kristin, who lived locally, went home. While I am glad that I stayed, seeing my father wheeled out in a body bag is a vision I can never, ever shake.

The following day, as I drove with my sister Sue to the cemetery to select a plot, I had to pull over when my husband called to tell me that the doctors felt fairly certain I had brain cancer. After several minutes, I continued driving to the cemetery, but I let my sisters handle the details of the arrangements. Sitting in the office of a cemetery is pretty much the LAST place you want to be ten minutes after you get a *terminal* cancer diagnosis!! I sat in the parking lot and cried until I had no more tears. All that ran through my mind was *How could this be happening to my children? How could life be THIS unfair?* Not one word of this account is an exaggeration. This shit truly went down. Once again, I pulled it together when we drove through the cemetery to view possible plots. I desperately wanted to honor my father by being a part of this final process and I did select the plot, one under a tree. My father loved trees.

Later that day, the spinal tap headaches hit. A spinal tap headache is caused by leaking spinal fluid. It is similar to a bad migraine headache. The only relief I felt was when I was lying down flat, which is hard to do when you are in the process of planning your father's funeral. I had to run out of the funeral director's conference room as I was ready to vomit from sitting upright. I had to leave picking the casket and the flowers to my sisters because I could not be upright at all. I did all this while still trying to convince my mother that I was having headaches due to grief. I drove back to my parents' house alone, one of the stupidest driving decisions of my life as I was dizzy, in terrible pain, and nauseous.

I wrote my father's eulogy lying on my back. I had moments of being okay, but after thirty minutes or so, I would have no choice but to lie down. My father died on a Wednesday, but the wake wasn't until Sunday night. We were all in the throes of grief and doing everything we could to muddle through.

I sent out a plea to God to allow me to stand throughout my father's wake to honor him. I was so concerned about this—I hadn't been able to stand or sit upright for more than thirty minutes for days—that I pulled the funeral director aside to arrange a signal with him if I needed to escape quietly to lie down without drawing too much attention. Miraculously, I was able to stand for five hours, without even a bathroom break, to greet and thank every person who came to pay their respects. I learned a lot about my father from the stories people shared. We only really know people from their relationship with us. I knew him as my father. At the wake, I got to know him as a high school kid, colleague, and friend. I learned how deeply respected he was for his integrity, a wonderful lasting impression.

I was also able to summon the strength to proceed through the funeral without too much pain. The reception, however, was hellishly uncomfortable. Several times I ducked out to lie down, but I tried to be there to honor my father. Almost no one knew what I was going through, which made it doubly difficult when at least two of my mother's friends pulled me aside to tell me that I must stay in Albany awhile longer to help my mother cope. While I appreciated their love for my mother, I knew that if I didn't get home and decompress in my own bed soon they would be using the plot next to my father's for me.

21

Once home, I began the process of accepting condolences from my Massachusetts friends. I began to hate flowers for what they now represented. I hated everything and simply wanted to disappear into the ether. I kept hoping the spinal tap headaches would go away, but the bastards kept coming back day after day. Five days after the funeral, I finally went to the pain clinic at the hospital where the most amazing doctor gave me an epidural patch.

Everyone I told my circumstance to felt tremendous pity for me, which honestly felt really good. When someone receives a new diagnosis, usually they receive a lot of support. In my case, as it coincided with my father's passing and I had a desire to protect my mother from my news, I had to comfort myself. The nurse in the pain clinic prayed with me and gave me a medal of Mary of Medjugorje. The doctor, a very kind man who couldn't believe I was given a spinal tap without pain management, delivered me almost immediate, once elusive, relief. It took effect quickly and I cried tears of peace for the first time in over a year. Once again I drove myself home, this time against doctors' orders because my husband had used up so much personal time with my father's funeral and my doctor's visits that I couldn't ask him to take more time off. This time, however, I was truly fine to drive.

I began writing thank you notes, planning my children's joint birthday party (complete with exotic animals), while continuing with doctor's appointments. On my son's birthday, I was able to get an appointment with a respected neurologist. I remember waiting for the neurologist at the hospital while his intern talked to him about my case. She didn't close the door, and I could hear him saying things like "disease progression" in relation to the numbness I was experiencing on my right side. I had only begun experiencing numbness *after* the cancer was found. Symptoms like numbness can be directly attributed to stress. The numbness intensified rapidly from my right arm to my right leg and even the right side of my face. I turned to my husband, Mike, and said, "This isn't good".

I moved to the big guns at the Dana Farber Cancer Center and Massachusetts General Hospital. Everywhere I went, the diagnosis was the same. When I finally found myself in a tiny, windowless room at the Dana Farber Cancer Center, my oncologist told me, "I know this is really shitty, but it gets better". It was the truest thing he ever said to me. I know he meant that I would learn to live with my condition until my untimely passing, but for me it was a beacon of hope, a moment that signaled *you are more than this diagnosis.*

The tumor could not be removed by surgery. It was too close to my speech center, and God bless him, my neurosurgeon did not want to create disability when I was experiencing no speech problems. Instead, I was scheduled for a small craniotomy in which a four-inch incision would be made and a large sample taken to determine definite diagnosis and staging. I had this done on Friday, August 13, 2010, yes indeed Friday the 13th! I wasn't really scared. I was numb.

The night before my surgery, my father visited me in my dream. Some might think it was just a dream, but I know better. Those on the other side often use dreams to communicate because our conscious minds are at rest and therefore less resistant to things we perceive as irrational. In the dream, my father and I were walking down Boylston Street in Boston. He was wearing his favorite red V-neck sweater and navy blue pants. In the next frame, I saw him across the street walking into an old Romanesque church. I tried to scream for him not to go in, but he went in anyway. The next thing I knew, I saw him being wheeled out of the church in a body bag and, in my dream, I began to crumble. A flash later, he was back at my side saying to me, "Erin, I didn't leave. I never leave". This is the only time my father has come in my dreams. When I woke before 5:00 a.m. the next morning to go to the hospital, I knew that he was with me.

I was a rock star patient. I was told I would be hospitalized for about three to four days. Once I was out of recovery and settled in the neuro ICU, I made it my mission to get the hell out of Dodge. The Neuro ICU at Brigham and Women's Hospital was set up like a traditional circular ICU with all glass doors. Every patient's head was wrapped in turban-style dressings. Everyone was unconscious except for me. I spent the night alone and terrified. My catheter was accidentally pulled partially out by a nurse who'd tripped, but I couldn't bear the thought of having it reinserted so I silently dealt with the discomfort. I also developed a blood sugar problem due to the steroids and required insulin injections in my abdomen. I wanted to go home. I was told that I needed to pass a series of tests to be discharged. I needed to eat, drink, walk the length of the ICU circle, climb a flight of stairs, and pee on my own. There is nothing like a little incentive to motivate you and I wanted out. Game on. The hardest one was peeing, simply because ICU rooms didn't have bathrooms. I had to resort to using a pull-down toilet (like a Murphy bed toilet) in my room.

I was discharged twenty-seven hours after my surgery. That was two hours later than it could have been, but it was a Saturday and I had to wait for the right neurosurgeon to make his rounds. I am still very proud of my determination.

The transition home wasn't seamless. One problem I encountered was the near-round-the-clock pills I had to take. I don't remember them all, but I had high doses of steroids for the brain swelling that made me jittery and exhausted at the same time. For several days, I was taking well over sixty pills a day. I hate steroids…

It felt good to be home, but it almost felt like having a baby without the joy of the baby—I seemed to always have a house full of people. I spent a lot of time in my bedroom just watching mind-numbing TV and letting the clock tick by. After about two weeks, I received the definite diagnosis: grade II astrocytoma. It was slow-growing, incurable brain cancer.

That was the last of me being the good little agreeable patient. Radiation was not offered yet as it led to brain damage and the oncologist thought I had more time. I turned down chemotherapy and started down the road less traveled. My father gave me the courage to do this because I witnessed his horrific suffering with chemotherapy and refused to do that to myself or my family when my doctors were telling me it wouldn't cure me and couldn't even say it would definitively extend my life. This is the part where people get scared of my approach sometimes, but I ask you, is it logical to follow a path that leads to certain death? I honestly believe logic was on my side even if conventional "wisdom" was not.

A friend of mine suggested that I see Dr. Mark Mincolla, a natural health practitioner. I figured I had nothing to lose. My first appointment with Dr. Mincolla was about a month after my surgery. Primarily through energetic, personalized nutrition, Dr. Mincolla has helped other people heal from brain cancer as well as other cancers, Lupus, diabetes, rheumatoid arthritis and heart disease. Dr. Mincolla listened to me, expressed his condolences over the loss of my father, and then handed me an article that gave me great confidence in him. The article was entitled "Cancer Is a Fungus."

My husband and I had had several conversations since my diagnosis about what might have caused the tumor. I knew that my stress and inability to effectively deal with my grief over my dad's illness played a huge part, even though doctors might not think so. I also knew my penchant for Crystal Lite lemonade with aspartame and my addiction to slightly burned microwave popcorn—both of which have been linked to brain tumors—surely didn't help. I also smoked in my twenties. Fungus (yeast) loves all this stuff, including the stress. We both suspected that it was also related to my poor health from a few years prior. *I was a red-hot mess.* I was pretty excited to read this article and approach healing from a different perspective, a perspective that actually felt like healing rather than poisoning myself.

Several years before my diagnosis, I had experienced a series of small medical fires that conventional doctors could not explain nor extinguish. It all started when I went on a birth control pill after the birth of my daughter, Kyra. At thirty-four, I had never had a yeast infection. Within six months of starting the pill, I had three plus three bouts of bacterial vaginosis. I also went through three weeks of irritable bowel syndrome where I could not leave my house—over the summer with kids, mind you—a rash on my hands that the dermatologist said was yeast, and a tooth that died out of the blue and required a root canal. I had been going to my dentist every six months for cleanings since I was a child. What was happening? My primary care doctor told me the bacterial vaginosis was unrelated to the yeast infections and were unrelated to the pill, the rash on my hands, my irritable bowel issues, and my tooth. I knew she was wrong.

With the help of Google, I diagnosed myself with a systemic yeast infection where yeast, which naturally lives in balance in the gut, grows out of control. I asked that my birth control prescription be lowered, and when it was, my problems, while never fully resolved, went from acute to low-grade chronic. *Never underestimate the power of your intuition.* Along with stress and antibiotics, one of the biggest triggers of systemic yeast infections is artificial hormones, but at that time at least, many conventionally-trained doctors wouldn't believe that, including my own.

Dr. Mincolla put me on a strict diet free of sugar, red meat, alcohol (*gulp*), dairy, and anything fermented. I also got the AMAS blood test, a Medicare-approved cancer screening, that could detect active cancer far earlier than MRIs or PET scans. My result came back positive for cancer, but a not very aggressive one, which coincided with my biopsy result. About a week after I began my diet, I experienced my first (and worst) of many detox reactions where so many pathogens were dying off that I felt like I had the flu. That's what happens when you finally begin to starve the microscopic invaders in your body. They die en masse and overload your elimination pathways. It lasted for a few hours.

I continued with my diet and rechecked my AMAS the following month. Unfortunately, my numbers went in the wrong direction, so Dr. Mincolla began adding supplements to fortify my immune system. He also told me that the pain I had felt in my chest a year earlier (when my father was at his weakest from chemotherapy) that my doctor dismissed as musculoskeletal pain was likely my thymus gland shouting out to me that the strain I was under was deeply damaging my immune system. After another month on the diet with supplements and now the addition of a Raindrop Treatment using Young Living essential oils to detoxify my body, my AMAS score landed me the very best noncancerous AMAS score Dr. Mincolla had ever seen. Anything under one hundred was considered normal. Mine was a twelve. Yeah, baby!

I continued to get AMAS tests on a regular basis along with MRIs. Health is fluid, not static. With the exception of two blips in three years (one after introducing a potent fungus detoxifier that overloaded my system again and the other after recovering from painful inflammation from dental surgery), my numbers were always normal, meaning no cancer. For the remainder of this book, because I have chosen to take a hiatus, possibly permanent, from checking the status of the tumor with MRIs, I will refer to the brain tumor in the present tense. This is not because I see it as a problem, but because it is easier for readers. I see the tumor as a benign reminder of my state of being. It is just a thing like any other. It can be there, be a part of my life, without having to control me or scare me.

I began to believe in my recovery, but I was still reliant on others to heal me. Although I was following a holistic path, I still didn't trust myself or my judgment. Three years into this journey, I hit a major roadblock that threatened to derail me. At an oncology appointment, my oncologist told me that he thought the tumor had grown by five millimeters. He said it was time for chemotherapy. I told him no. He questioned my sanity. I agreed to come back three months later for a follow-up.

Those three months were terrible. I felt scared and lost. I had almost no one to turn to except my husband, one friend, and Dr. Mincolla. Everyone else in my life, had I revealed what the oncologist had said, would have pushed me into chemotherapy out of fear. If you don't have the right support, go forward on your own. Misguided, fear-based support can be very detrimental. I had to stay quiet and once again suffer in silence. My nerves got so bad that my numbness returned. Luckily, Dr. Mincolla suggested a supplement, vinpocetine, to calm my *nervous* system. It worked within two hours without side effects. The numbness was gone.

At the follow-up MRI, my oncologist, a good guy, came in beaming and said, "Great news, there's been no growth, and after reviewing the scans over the last eighteen months, I am confident in saying that it hasn't grown". You see, several of my MRIs had been taken at different facilities. That alone can account for the changes because MRIs are still reliant on a radiologist's interpretation, which can be wrong. I also concede that from my first MRI in June 2010 until I got the tumor under control in November 2010 there could have been growth. When my oncologist shared this good news with me, I wanted to throw a brick at him. Did he have any idea the agony he had put me through in the last three months? Instead I said to him (pretty damn nicely under the circumstances), "It's a good thing I didn't listen to you three months ago when you erroneously told me to start chemotherapy". That was the last MRI I had.

Some may call my decisions crazy, but what is the point of checking in on something that cannot be healed conventionally? Doesn't that just perpetuate a feeling of helplessness and fear? Anybody who has been through the cancer screening process knows how terrifying the buildup to scans and the wait for results can be. You feel powerless. Beyond that, the cycle of nervous tension is highly toxic to my body and mind. I am not advocating for others to do the same—I wouldn't want that responsibility—I am simply explaining that *I* chose to focus on living, not on a condition that conventional medicine itself told me was incurable. Why did I have to continue to play by those rules? It was time to turn the page if I ever wanted to be free.

Had I started chemotherapy, which, in case you didn't realize, is a *known carcinogen*, there is a good chance I wouldn't be writing this today. Yes, I chose a different path. Yes, it's a path that makes some people uncomfortable, but why would I invest in a system that was practically guaranteed to eventually fail me? If I did that, it would only be out of fear. Decisions made in fear are rarely for my highest good.

I know several people who have healed brain cancer naturally. I know many more who have healed other cancers naturally. We don't hear about them very often. Why do you think that is? I think it might have something to do with the fact that cancer is big business. Between the enormous state-of-the-art cancer centers, cancer charities, and pharmaceutical profit margins, if someone said clean eating and a healthy mind could cure you, what would happen to this business? Beyond that, pharmaceutical companies have a monopoly on network news advertising. Are they really going to allow a segment on natural cancer cures on the same broadcast as their advertisements for drugs to help erectile dysfunction and psoriasis? I don't think so. I knew this, but had it hammered home to me after reading Billy Best's[2] autobiography in which he shares how he healed from leukemia without chemotherapy.

Billy Best was a Massachusetts teen who ran away from home in the 1990s to avoid chemotherapy after watching his aunt suffer and die from chemotherapy and cancer. He was a national news celebrity. He returned home only when his parents agreed that he wouldn't be forced to have chemotherapy. He healed himself by using a supplement that he illegally smuggled in from Canada. The NBC affiliate in Boston wanted to do a follow-up piece on him after he healed, only for the reporter to call him the day before it was due to air saying that the story had been killed—in her opinion because it ruffled too many feathers among pharmaceutical advertisers. That's a true story. You can find his book on Amazon.

Cancer is being healed naturally every day. My test results have been so good that if I actually went for a scan the tumor might be gone, but even if it is still there, what's the big deal? A tumor is just a shell that the immune system builds around toxicity. Many people have cancer and they don't even know it. For a lot of these people, the body heals the cancer without them ever knowing they had it. If it goes away I will be pleased. If it stays I will live with it and learn from it. If ultimately some day I die from it, then it was part of my soul's journey. I don't know the future. I know the now. I was given the gift of presence because I was reminded that the life journey always has an end. It has an end for all of us. That's why it is a gift to me. It is my reminder and can be yours too. What will you do with your now knowing that tomorrow might not be?

I have had to learn to rely on my intuition more than anyone else, no matter their credentials. My purification brings me closer to my soul purpose. It hasn't been an easy journey; a trial by fire is pretty hot and uncomfortable. It is what I needed to kick my ass into gear and embrace my power. I have absolutely no idea when I will check out of this life, but I don't think it will be anytime soon. I expect to be around to see my children get married and to snuggle with my grandchildren, but I honestly don't know. That makes me the same as you. Today could be my last day or your last day. It is what we do with today that matters because that is where we have power. I am learning to trust my own inner wisdom and to listen for advice that feels right to me on a deep level. I have a couple of methods to check in on the state of my health, but for the most part, I focus on what I want, not on what I don't, one of my key insights for living an inspired life. Sometimes I get frustrated. Sometimes I get angry, but I never feel that life is unfair because I know that God brings me gifts in every form, even if the packaging is downright terrifying to my human perception.

I am a far better person for this experience. I continue to focus on my good health: to make decisions about what I eat, drink, and do that are for my highest good. I am a much better mother now that I have come to love myself because I can finally teach my children to love themselves. I am a better wife, a better friend, and love sharing inspiration wherever I go. We each create the lives that we live, and we each have power to change how we feel about what we get. I encourage you to suck the nectar out of every opportunity or challenge that comes your way.

We all fear the unknown. We all fear illness. I do not blame myself or anyone else for their illness. In fact, I generally don't see illness as a curse, but as an opportunity. I am very concerned when I hear people say that getting cancer, diabetes, heart disease, or rheumatoid arthritis is just bad luck or genetics. While that might make the patient feel less responsible, it also takes their power to change and heal away from them. I sincerely believe that illness is one of the most powerful tools the soul can use to grow. I would never expect you to jump for joy at a new, scary-sounding diagnosis, but I hope that you can open yourself, your heart, and your soul to the experience. You will learn more from your challenges then you could ever learn without them.

Does that mean that every illness is caused by emotional turmoil? I doubt it. I think genetics predisposes people to various illnesses, and what we eat, drink, and inhale affects our health, but I also believe that something is triggering the expression of our predispositions—an X factor—and I think it is often emotional wounds, stress, or a feeling of being disconnected from a larger meaning in life. Someone can have a seemingly ideal life, but be in turmoil inside. Inner storms manifest outwardly eventually.

My perspective on almost everything has changed simply because of one or two, the MRI could never determine, white matter lesion.

Perspective is a powerful force with the ability to change the way our world appears to us. Some people assume that a person with Down Syndrome has a disability worth aborting. Others know someone with Down Syndrome who finds joy in every moment, relishes the simplest experiences that most of us overlook, and loves with no self-consciousness. Your experience is what you make of it.

Lastly, I want you to know how imperfectly perfect I am. I eat way more veggie chips than my holistic practitioner would sanction. Sometimes I yell at my kids. Sometimes I don't want any lessons. I am human. I make mistakes, get in bad moods, and most definitely don't always do the right thing. Life is a paradox. Knowing things with certainty is the surest way to get bitch-slapped by life. I am now at a place where I value humility much more than mastery because mastery inevitably leads to defending a position against that other person who has mastered the opposite view! Convincing others to agree with your opinion is just an ego game even if you think it is the worthiest cause.

I chose to call these chapters *Phoenix Burning* and *Phoenix Rising* after the great bird of Greek mythology that rose from the ashes and was reborn. I have most definitely been transformed for the better for all that I have experienced on this journey. I am no expert on life, and honestly, I think we could all use a little less proselytizing. I have simply uncovered some great pearls of wisdom that have enriched my life, and I want to share them with you. I don't take credit for these insights more than I was the right soul at the right time in the right predicament to bring them forth. The following chapters are twenty-five pearls of wisdom I have learned by living my life with an expanded perspective due to a little tumor in my head. A lot of what I have discovered is actually *unlearning* dogma that has been engrained in us by government, formal education, religion, and parents, and other experts passed down generation to generation, and instead reconnecting with the wisdom inside of us. I hope these insights encourage you to question your conditioning and inspire you to believe that you were meant to thrive and live out a purpose designed *souly* for you.

1.

Vibration is Your Signature Scent

Once you make a decision, the universe conspires to make it happen.

Ralph Waldo Emerson

God loves you so much that He wants you to be successful in everything. Everything in the universe is energy. This journey in life is a partnership with the Divine so whatever signal you are sending out will be met with more evidence of the same. That works amazingly well when you are sending out winning signals such as "I am successful" or "I am healthy" but it also works for the person who sends out "I am worried" or "I am a mess".

When scientists look at atoms under a microscope, they discover that at their core there is just a vibrating tornado of energy. We are made of atoms. That means we are energy at our core even though we look and feel solid. We emit our own energy signal. We feel our own and other people's signals, too. It's how we make decisions about whom we associate with. When someone shares a similar vibration, we want to be closer to them. When someone's vibration is far different, we are repelled.

Every feeling, event, and activity has an energy vibration. Our job is matching our vibration to that which we wish to attract, just like setting a radio dial to the station we want. We are like radio transmitters and receivers to the universe pinging out signals all day long. Just like a radio, whatever frequency (measure of vibration) we are tuned to is what we are going to experience. If you want to listen to Top 40, tuning in to the classic rock station's frequency is not going to get you there. It's not personal. It's not about deserving it. It is simply the result of the station you are tuned to.

Where does your dominant vibration come from? I have studied and pondered this a lot in the last several years. I do not have definitive proof of the answer, but I have my beliefs. Plastic surgeon Dr. Maxwell Maltz[3] suggests that our self-image sets the vibrational channel that we are tuned to. This is something that we develop in childhood and spend our adult years reinforcing, for good or bad. Do you see yourself as more of a success or more of a failure? Do things work out easily, or do you face challenge after challenge? Do you see others as smarter than you? Do you believe you are an attractive person? Do you like you? You are setting your vibration with each perception about yourself.

The good news is that you can change your vibration in every moment. Energy vibration is fluid, not static. I can bring myself lower with a little bitching about a common complaint, jealousy, or by judging others. Modern society is actually powerfully tuning us to low vibration. Feeling bad, scared, and stressed is addictive. Just look at the TV and movie entertainment we choose and the *news* programs we watch. Do they make your body feel good or bad? Really think about your answer to that question…

I have found that I have to be very careful about visiting my past because many of those people don't see me as *well*. They remember me from long ago when I was a far different person, or they have heard I am *sick* and determine to see me as what they perceive a sick person looks and acts like. They don't realize how much I have changed and project an image of me that is no longer true. They struggle to understand how I can have the diagnosis I do, but look healthier than they do. I find that I avoid doctors in social settings too because most have their stations set to *not well*, looking for the diseases that people have. I have been derailed by doctors in social settings tilting their heads slightly while sympathetically offering a "how are you?" I get why they do it. In the medical world, very few people are well. We cover symptoms with drugs, but generally don't cure them. Most doctors are also not well trained in emotional health and how dramatically it impacts the physiology of the body and therefore sometimes lack sensitivity. They are also used to being around patients who feel like victims, patients who are used to being reminded of their frailties.

While circumstances can bring me lower, I am still responsible for my vibration. Each external challenge is just another opportunity for me to reaffirm my desired state of being, reaffirm my self-image. It's like a little test asking us "how bad do you want it?" I can bring my vibration up quickly. A ten-minute meditation, a funny video, or five minutes in nature all work well and easily. My vibration affects that of my family, even the dogs. Recently I even noticed that my dear friend's baby son starts to hold his head in pain when she and I (a friend in tune with energy vibration) start to discuss something of a low vibration. He literally breaks up our conversations when they are low. Babies, young children, and animals are often highly attuned to energy vibration.

Sometimes, we are in sync with someone. "We are on the same wavelength", we say. When odd coincidences occur, we call them synchronicities. Do you ever get a bad vibe from someone? Have you ever noticed how your mood changes when someone in a bad mood walks in the room?

Do our vibrational buttons get pushed by others? You bet. Are they responsible for our vibration? No. It's our perception not reality that matters. I can respond to their vibrational issue any way I choose. Don't blame your boss, your spouse, or the guy who cut you off in traffic. Yes, they triggered a reaction in you, but you are responsible for how you feel and the button-pushers are actually challenging you to choose better reactions. You have free will. Each trigger is an opportunity to continue with your set station or to change the channel.

We are energetic beings with an electromagnetic field around our bodies. This energy is often called *chi*, or *life force* energy. In fact, a couple of years ago, I began seeing this energy field around some people. To me it looks like a pale yellow halo around the entire body. I am particularly able to see it when the lighting is low and the person is feeling centered, which raises their energy vibration. The first time this happened I was with a group of very spiritually connected women

35

at a meditation. I began noticing it on myself and others, too. I don't see them all the time, only on those with a high vibration and only when my vibration is high, too, which isn't every moment of every day!

Have you noticed that the wealthy tend to stay wealthy and the poor tend to stay poor? It's not about deserving wealth. I wish the Kardashians no harm, but clearly they don't deserve their prosperity any more than the volunteer at the women's shelter does. I believe it is about their self-image, the energy vibration that they are pinging out. To consistently emit a vibration, the way to turn vibration into matter, you must first be familiar with the feeling of that vibration. Someone like Donald Trump has consistently known wealth, so even when he has gone through bankruptcies he is familiar enough with the feeling (vibration) of prosperity that he can tap into it again easily. I realize that he takes action as well, but it is action with intention and belief in himself. The opposite is true for the blue-collar worker who wins the lottery and winds up penniless again soon after. He doesn't know the feeling of wealth enough to keep pinging it. He is far more accustomed to the *I am poor* vibration or self-image, his preset station.

This same principle can be applied to disease. Life experiences, particularly traumatic events, have a profound effect on our vibration. An RN from the Dana Farber Cancer Center even shared with me that fifty percent of the patients she saw had experienced a significant trauma, shock, or loss in the three years preceding their diagnosis. While it's anecdotal, I find it significant. I have also read many books on holistic cancer healing. They consistently highlight the emotional element in the formation of disease. If you ping out *I'm anxious*, you'll experience more to be anxious about. If you ping out *I'm afraid I'll get sick*, you draw *sick* closer to you. I am a real world example of both. Once my father was diagnosed with lung cancer, not only did I become consumed with researching treatments for him, but I also got nervous for myself. I smoked in my twenties. I was aware of predisposition to disease, and I knew my chances of getting cancer just went up. Cancer became my obsession for eleven months BEFORE my diagnosis. *I vibrated my dominant fear.*

I do not believe that disease just happens. One of the great gaps in our health care, in my opinion, is how we fail to address mental and emotional feelings, self-esteem, and the enormous contribution they make to our health. Lifestyle can certainly play a part, as can genetics, but I consider stress one of the biggest lifestyle threats. Breast cancer has been linked to a lack of nurturing: either of the self, issues with mother figures, or not having the opportunity to nurture others. Lung cancer has been linked to grief, of which Dana Reeve, the nonsmoking wife of Christopher Reeve, is an example. Brain cancer has been linked to overthinking and refusing to change old patterns. Damn, I can relate...

Many of us get stuck on a particular station. I was stuck on the not good enough blues for a long time. My station was set as a child, just like many of us. Even though I heard snippets of what the other stations were playing, I just couldn't seem to keep my tuner dial from reverting back to what it always knew—until I was given an opportunity to change my station via disease. Disease is a powerful messenger from the soul, a station-changing opportunity for those who see it.

If you talked to the patients who achieve lasting remission, you might discover that beyond their treatments they also began to listen to the message of their disease and made the life changes that were crying out to them, things they had been too afraid to do before disease manifested. These are the people who quit their life-sucking jobs, went on the dream trip, got a pet, and generally stopped waiting for life to get better and instead decided to *make* it better. These are the people who changed their vibrational stations. Is their healing a result of the treatments or the change in their perspective?

I am a big believer in *fake it till you make it*. No matter what you are yearning for in life, begin to act as if you have already achieved your goal—that's an effective way to change the station. Your perception *is* your reality. Are you perceiving success or failure? Are you perceiving health or disease? Use phrases like *I AM healed*, *I AM happy*, *I AM prosperous*, in the present tense. Use a journal, EFT (tapping on acupressure points to release harmful patterns), or affirmations. If you are very down, you might not have an immediate transformation in your attitude. You can, but sometimes it takes patience. Just keep practicing. If you long ago wired yourself to see obstacles, you might need practice adjusting your view to see opportunities, but if I can do it, you surely can! Make sure your feelings' tuner dial is set to the station you want to experience with no static. The universe will respond to your dominant vibration and deliver you more that matches. Your station is an excellent indicator of the kind of future you are attracting.

2.

The Body is a Biofeedback System

So often times it happens, that we live our lives in chains, and we never even know we have the key.

The Eagles

The body is the vehicle we travel in to experience the game of life. There are no accidents from the cosmic perspective. Most people are beginning to realize that allergies are overreactions of our immune systems. Stress creates ulcers. Constipation creates headaches. The body is always trying to communicate with us.

Emotions are messages. They are meant to be energy in motion—*e-motion,* not meant to be stored within us for all eternity! I have often read that emotions are like the weather. They don't stay with us permanently, and we have little control over them. If you are anything like me, you may believe that hiding your emotions in many instances is an admirable quality. It is a revered trait among modern cultures. In fact, two of the characteristics of those who develop cancer are stoicism and the habit of pushing through and getting by. Often, those who develop cancer are seen as the steady ones. Throughout my life, I harbored self-loathing, never displaying it outwardly, but carrying it like a parasite in my body. The final straw came with my father's cancer diagnosis when my biofeedback system basically yelled, "Holy shit, if we don't give her a loud and clear signal, she is never going to change!" Enter the brain tumor.

When my father was at a very weak point due to his first-line chemotherapy treatment, he told me, "Erin, I'm dying". It broke my heart. This was many months before he actually passed away, but the effects of chemotherapy were so profoundly toxic to his body that he felt that all his cells were dying. I tried to tell him that it was the effects of the chemotherapy, not the cancer, that was making him feel like that, but he didn't believe me. In fact, he felt perfectly fine before he started chemotherapy. After just six weeks of treatment, he was in that wretched state.

A few days later, I woke up with a searing pain in the center of my chest. I couldn't breathe deeply or stretch. I went to my primary care doctor, thinking I might have pneumonia. The doctor listened to my chest, told me it was musculoskeletal pain, and suggested I not stretch the area until the pain cleared. Our energetic heart, directly in the center of the breast bone, is associated with the thymus gland of the endocrine system. The thymus gland regulates the release of powerful immune system cells whose job is to seek out and destroy cancerous cells in the body.

It would be beneficial if some of the paperwork we fill out before seeing doctors asked questions about emotional and mental stress and not just physical complaints. They are powerfully connected. The pain continued, but having listened to my doctor, I simply didn't stretch out, further constricting my heart energy. Only after I started working with a natural health practitioner did I realize that my heart center was providing me with a very loud alarm that my immune system could not keep up with the immense stress of my father's illness. My broken heart was profoundly affecting my body's ability to self-regulate.

I no longer feel the pain in my chest. It took at least two years, maybe more, before I consistently got to a place where thumping on my chest did not hurt. Now I know that if that area feels tender, I need to treat myself with love and practice activities that are stress relieving. I need to acknowledge and honor the feelings, positive or negative, that are working their way through me rather than constrict myself and hold my pain inside.

Louise Hay, noted self-help author, compiled a list of likely emotional and mental patterns that contribute to various diseases and conditions in *Heal Your Body*.[4] I highly recommend it to help you to understand why you get the messages that you do. I have taken some of my *issues* from the past to highlight the emotional element that likely led to it. Enjoy my dirty laundry...

<u>Menstrual Problems</u>: Rejection of one's femininity. Guilt, fear. Belief that the genitals are sinful or dirty.

<u>Yeast</u>: Denying your own need. Not supporting yourself.

<u>Spastic Colitis</u>: Fear of letting go. Insecurity.

<u>Root Canal</u>: Can't bite into anything anymore. Root beliefs being destroyed.

<u>Cancer</u>: Deep hurt. Longstanding resentment. Deep secret or grief eating away at the self. Carrying hatreds. "What's the use?"

And last but not least...<u>Brain Tumor</u>: Incorrect computerized beliefs. Stubborn. Refusing to change old patterns.

We all have hidden pain. You don't need to write a book to broadcast yours, but I hope you will begin to honor the messages you are getting and love yourself for exactly who you are, accepting your pain and the parts of yourself that your ego decided were *unworthy*.

Yes, what we eat and drink impacts our health. Yes, there are biological reactions taking place that cause heart disease, cancer, and arthritis pain, but why stop there? Why aren't we asking the obvious question: why did the biological reactions start? Genetics is a pat answer to a complicated question. Expression of genes seems to be at least partially controlled by lifestyle factors, including emotional well-being.

Ultimately, every symptom is just an indication that your being is out of balance. Even pharmaceutical companies rarely speak of curing a disease. They focus on managing it. When someone has a disease, the focus should be on restoring balance (homeostasis) in the body, not on eliminating symptoms. The labels that modern medicine uses keep us focused on solving the symptom rather than on getting balanced, which is all the body wants to do! Sure, you can take the medicine to make the infection go away, but why did it come in the first place?

Fulfilled people are healthier. I wish that wasn't my conclusion because it feels like piling on people who already have heavy burdens, but it is what I have found to be true. I had to work at accepting myself, and when I did, my body responded beautifully. The more fulfilled I have become—in all my messy humanness—the healthier I have become.

The human body has an amazing self-repair mechanism designed to heal everything from cuts and scrapes to cancer, but it only works when the body feels relaxed and safe. Sadly, modern living keeps us in a near-constant state of stress. We all know it as fight or flight, and we probably also know that we produce extra cortisol (aka the death hormone) when we are stressed. The amygdala, responsible for emotions, survival instinct and memory in the brain, doesn't know the difference between real and imaginary threats—running from that tiger versus worrying someone else might get your promotion. Stress throws the body out of homeostatic balance and prevents healing. Is it any wonder how many people develop cancer after a life trauma such as a loved one developing cancer?

I look back on the last weeks of my father's life and the first weeks of my diagnosis and am disappointed that doctors were prescribing me antianxiety and antidepressant medications. While I appreciate their attempt to lighten my burden, why was it not okay for me to be a mess under those extraordinarily difficult circumstances? I was managing okay. I was getting out of bed every day, getting dressed and looking after my kids. I was not falling apart. Dulling the pain simply *represses* it. Pain is natural, it's life, and it is the most direct path so that the pain doesn't get stuck to me. The very best assistance that I received came from the grief counselor who simply listened to me.

When a child is afraid of the monster in the closet, do you dismiss her concerns, scream at her, tell her she is stupid, or drug her? Of course not! And yet, when you feel scared, jealous, or angry, you beat yourself up for it, ignore it, drug it, or lock it away. There is nothing wrong with those feelings. Really, there isn't. Just like the monster in the closet, the very best remedy for scary feelings is light.

The next time you feel bad, whether it is a headache or a subtle feeling of jealousy, shine a light on it. Accept that it was brought to you on purpose, as everything is, to teach you something, and allow it to pass over you without attaching to it. Keep a journal, draw, scream, or do whatever calls to you, just let that shit out and ease your burden. Appreciate that you created it at a higher level of consciousness to help you clear a limiting belief that you have probably lived with since early childhood, when the seeds of many of our lies and limitations were planted by our egos misconstruing external events. Appreciate how powerful you are to have created this lesson and opportunity for growth. Ask it what it wants you to know and wait for the subtle reply that pops into your awareness. Soothe it just like you would a scared child. Just like a child, once it feels like it has been seen and heard (and appreciated), the feeling will calm down.

As I began to do this, I no longer strove for answers to my healing. Life became far easier simply because I realized that everything showing up for me was for my benefit, even if I didn't understand why. I appreciate my biofeedback system and the way it keeps me connected with my soul.

3.

I Remembered God

This is my commandment, that you love one another as I have loved you.

Jesus Christ

God never abandoned me. I had lost contact with Him/Her/Me for many years. The religion I participated in did not work for me because it made me believe God was outside of me. Religion offers a beautiful community of spiritually-minded people; however, I could not thrive in a system that asked me not to question, not to come up with my own interpretation of God. Every religion believes it is the one true religion, and every religion is a manmade institution, a human interpretation of God's will.

Most institutions are ripe with dogma, *incontrovertibly* true doctrine. We like this and accept it because it takes away our burden of discovering what is true for us. We assume it's the easier path, but is it? History has shown us time and again that nothing is beyond question or revision. Dogma changes from generation to generation. Unfortunately, history also shows that those who challenge the conventional dogma, although often proven right posthumously, suffer ridicule while alive.

Anybody who knows me knows that telling me I can't do something is the surest way to get me to try it. "You have an incurable cancer?" "Oh yeah? Watch me." When I was in college, I was very interested in Middle Eastern studies and announced to my parents my intention to study abroad in Lebanon. My parents were terrified, but wise as they were to how I operated, they said nothing to dissuade me. Had they tried, I would have spent my junior year in Lebanon instead of where I ended up, Oxford University in jolly old England.

Many people when they are diagnosed with a scary disease turn to their church. I think that is beautiful. I, too, sought counsel from my parish priest and even had the Anointing of the Sick sacrament. But as much as I tried, I just couldn't connect with the hierarchy and pageantry. Religion made me feel smaller. So after a short reconnection, I pulled away from organized religion again.

God reached out to me first on the day I said goodbye to my father at the hospital, the last day I saw him alive, when the young man ran up behind me to tell me "God asked me to tell you God bless you." God was still an external force to me at that point. What I have evolved to over these past few years is an awareness that if God created me, created you, created trees, oceans, planets, stars, and fire ants, then doesn't that mean that God is within all of us? To me, it also means that I am an aspect, a divine spark of God, and that I can, therefore, never be separated from Her. I experience God as the creative energy of the universe that I refer to as Divine Love. I don't believe that God is an old Caucasian man with a white beard. God is Divine Love, the energy of creation. It doesn't reward or punish, but responds to our vibration. I see my relationship with God as a partnership. Divine Love is the life force energy (physical and spiritual) that courses through my life delivering me opportunities that match my vibration.

I believe that God splintered into trillions of pieces to experience all there is from different perspectives. How exciting it would be to truly stand in another's shoes for a short time. That is what I believe we are all here doing. Helping God to play the game of life. When we were born, we signed on to play a role as a God particle, to feel life from a unique perspective. I believe the ultimate objective in life is not to achieve lofty goals, but to relish every minute of the experiences that our unique perspectives offer, not for all of us to conform to the same one.

I don't say that I found God, because I could never be separated from Her. She is me. She is you. *I remembered Her* when I started seeing God in nature, in people, and in events that once might have distressed me, but now I could observe their perfection from a higher perspective.

We are all connected by a vast web of energy (Divine Love), which is why mothers in New York can feel that something terrible has happened to their child in California. We are all one entity fractured into trillions of pieces. We need to treat one other with the respect that we would give a priest, a rabbi, or the President of the United States. Once a critical mass of humanity can begin to follow the wisdom of a great spiritual teacher, Jesus Christ, when he said, *Love one another as I have loved you*—one of the best aspects of my original faith— I believe our planet will experience a great awakening.

That awakening seems to be happening now. The Mayans did not predict the end of the world in December 2012. They predicted the end of a cycle, the end of a time of darkness. Even the word *apocalypse* has been distorted by world powers to denote doom, gloom, and to promote fear. The actual meaning of the ancient Greek word *apocalypse* is unveiling or revealing, as in the biblical book of Revelation.

I see the awakening happening in so many ways, but one fine example is the resignation of Pope Benedict XVI and the election of Pope Francis. Pope Benedict XVI seemed mired in the old guard of the Vatican. He promoted separation and secrecy. Pope Francis, who chose to emulate the humble St. Francis of Assisi in his official title, is broadcasting a message of love, inclusion, and care for our fellow humans. Pope Benedict was the first since Pope Gregory in 1415 to resign. A rather remarkable event!

I don't need to do anything or be anything other than the most authentic version of myself that I can attain every moment. In fact, I don't need to figure out how to heal myself at all. Divine Love clearly knows what is needed if I am meant to be healed. God created the universe; I'm pretty sure He can handle a tumor. I have learned to surrender to higher wisdom that my limited ego mind is not privy to. I have learned to surrender the heavy lifting to God and just ride the wave of life, open and aware.

4.

Reboot Before You Fry Your System

Life can be frustrating sometimes. Take a nap, exercise, meditate, or do whatever it takes to 'reboot' your thinking. Happiness is just a thought away!

Tom Giaquinto

Sometimes the shit really hits the fan. You get dealt a blow, and then another, and another. This pattern has happened to most, if not all, of us at one time or another. We try so hard to fix it, stop it, shield ourselves and our loved ones from it, and yet we still get sprayed with shit.

I have become the poster child for Helen Reddy's song "I Am Woman" these last few years, as in *wisdom born of pain*. As such, I have learned a few things. Struggling against forces of nature and the supernatural is futile. Whatever crisis has made its way to you is there for you to experience, and sometimes the best thing you can do is reboot your system before it's fried.

In the summer of 2010, my life as I knew it was crumbling around me. I lost my father and was diagnosed with a condition that I was told would kill me sooner rather than later. I am a mother. That immediately raised the stakes for me. It was a lot to handle in a nine-day period. Normally, my father and my husband would have been my rocks. My father was unavailable for this particular gig, and my husband was distraught at not only the loss of my dad, whom he adored, but the loss of me that he was already projecting. I didn't blame him. In some ways, I thought I had it easier than my husband because he was processing how he would pick up the pieces after I was gone. We had two young children (eight and five years old) that we were trying to protect, and we had no idea where to turn for help.

47

I was dealing with some crazy shit that not only included the loss of my dad and my new diagnosis, but also included telling my mother about my diagnosis two weeks after she lost my father, meeting countless neurologists and oncologists, getting second and third opinions, and connecting to everyone I knew in the medical field— while keeping my kids from appreciating the seriousness of the situation as they had just lost their beloved grandfather to cancer by throwing a double birthday party for thirty kids in my backyard complete with exotic animals (no joke). As if that wasn't enough, I was also scheduling and having brain surgery, recovering from it with high-dose steroids that made me jittery, exhausted, and yet unable to sleep, and reassuring family, friends, and priests that I was okay, because *you learn quickly* that no one, unless they have been through something similar, can help you. When your loved ones call or come by to check on you, you spend most of your time rehashing the same information and comforting them as they cry, and it's exhausting. The lowest moment may have been while talking on the phone with a lovely, compassionate priest and dear family friend, whose advice to me was that I needed to speed up the life education for my children while I was able.

Have you ever called the cable company when your box was on the fritz? The very first thing they tell you to do is to turn the box off and back on. Very technical solution, right? It's the first thing my husband (our family tech support) tells me to do if my phone bugs out, too. Pretty much every tech department uses this first line of defense. When the system gets fried, it's best to reboot.

You know what I did to get through my hellish summer? I watched hours of Everybody Loves Raymond, which happened to be on reruns. While it's an entertaining show, it isn't exactly riveting TV. I didn't want to think about anything, and that show let me just coast for a while. My dogs would lie on the bed with me while I half watched. That show gave me the breather I needed to handle each challenge as it arose.

I also did something very life affirming. I got another dog. I wasn't in the market for a dog—we already had two wonderful labrador retrievers—but this one dog had my heart months earlier. We were meant for each other.

For many months before my diagnosis, I took my kids to the pet store in the mall—which is now closed, thank God—to play with the dogs they were selling. I did it to socialize the dogs, for my kids to feel joy, and, who am I kidding, for me, too. For at least three months we saw a Shih Tzu. She was so loving and playful, and we adored her. The salesperson at the pet store told us she was being overlooked because she was getting older and people wanted puppies. This poor creature spent the first six months of her life in a cage, at first in the puppy mill where she was born and then in a pet store. Her price was continually dropped. When she was down to eight hundred dollars, I called my husband and asked if he'd be okay with me bringing home a third dog. This was about a month after my surgery. Bills were stacking up and stress levels were through the roof. He kindly told me he didn't think it would be a great idea, so I dropped it. One month later on a Tuesday in October, I was at the Borders bookstore, which happened to be across from the pet store. I decided to make sure the Shih Tzu had finally found a home, but when I walked in, there she was. Her price had been lowered that morning to four hundred dollars. I called my husband again and explained the situation. I told him it was "unlikely that I could walk out without this dog." He agreed. I bought a collar, a leash, a crate, and small-breed dog food. I told the salesperson that I needed to buy myself some joy, and that's just what I named her on the spot. Joy has seen me through some dark days. I rescued her, and she rescued me. She was a true gift from God at a time when I really needed something to lighten my load.

The best way to be clear when the storms are raging is to disconnect from the chaos for a time. Focus on what would bring you joy. If you can't reach joy from your state of despair, then what would bring you comfort or peace? Do that.

Don't explain yourself to anybody and don't feel like you need to be there for family and friends beyond your children. If it's a medical crisis, designate a friend or family member to be the fun maker for your kids or to be your communication point person to everyone else, but then take care of you. When things get tough in your life, your most important job is relieving your own stress. Stress creates and intensifies challenges. Take walks in nature, watch really funny movies, and spend time with people or animals that make you feel okay. Don't turn to alcohol or illicit or pharmaceutical drugs to change your mood. You need clarity, not cloudiness. Temporary distraction can be just what you need. Reboot your system in any way that elevates your energy vibration.

5.

<u>Don't Wait for Perfect Timing</u>

Don't wait. The time will never be just right.

Napoleon Hill

Maybe you have read about the wisdom of those on their deathbeds and what they want to share with us about what is really important. Perhaps you think you are too busy in the minutia of your daily life to pursue your dreams today. Maybe tomorrow you'll have more time.

What if there was no tomorrow? I don't mean to scare you. It's just that most of us live our days as if our lives will never end. If we really knew how fleeting life would be, we would never worry about anything, would we? Norman Vincent Peale reminds us that *the present is the gift*. I have come to embrace this as a very important spiritual truth.

When I got on this crazy roller coaster, I immediately began looking to the future. Looking is probably too kind of a word. A better word might be *obsessing*. "Would I have a future? Would my kids have a mother? Shit, this is it?" This is where my mind was in those first couple of months, which wasn't very productive whether I believed I could heal or not. When I began working with Dr. Mincolla, I had not heard of anybody surviving what I had—with or without conventional treatments—and yet somewhere in the deep recesses of my mind I had this unexplainable confidence that everything would be okay. Consciously, I hadn't reached that perspective yet, but it was there simmering and just waiting for external confirmation. Then I was told about people who were healing naturally; I started connecting with some of them and got excited! I was being given a second lease on life.

Unfortunately, I fell back into the pattern of living for the future almost immediately. I decided that all would be well *when I healed*. I could inspire others *when I healed*. I could share my story and write about the life lessons I am learning *when I healed*. I was not satisfied with simply living and being here now. I tied my happiness and my life purpose to proving that I could *beat* cancer. I spent at least three years in this state of waiting for my life to begin.

And then something shifted. I don't even know what triggered it, but one day I decided I didn't feel like waiting anymore; besides, without MRIs I wouldn't ever *officially* know if the tumor was gone, so why wait? I felt powerfully pulled to share what I am learning. I had wisdom to share that could really help people, so I started my blog. About a year later, I launched my professional Facebook page. I realized that *healed* is a state of being that had much more to do with my mind than my body. I might be cured, but I am not willing to get back on the fear train to find out, so I'll stay where I am for now.

No one can know what it feels like to be me on the inside, but I can tell you with certainty that my mind and body are well. When my mind is peaceful, the energy it transmits to my body makes my cells very happy. As my cells are happier, my body chemistry follows. I know when some people read that they assume I am delusional, and I know there is very little I can do to change their minds. That's okay, because I am no longer in the business of needing to change people's minds.

I still experience some numbness from time to time on the right side of my body when I am under more stress, a perfect message from my biofeedback system reminding me to slow down. The numbness happens less frequently than when I was first diagnosed, because I no longer live with monumental stress that accompanies the manic schedule of a new diagnosis's tests and appointments. I got off that particular ride and I began to thrive. I am far healthier mentally, emotionally, and physically than I ever was before.

I don't wait for the perfect conditions to live my life or pursue my dreams. I make the most of every moment I get. I have no idea when my hotel check out will be, and neither do you, but I intend to maximize my use of the facilities until hotel management has me escorted from the building.

Do you have any *everything will be good when…* scenarios? If that *when* never came to pass, would you be enough without it? The truth is that you already are enough. All you needed to do to prove your worth was to be born. Don't wait for perfect timing. Be the kind of person you admire…now.

6.

Solitude Unleashes Your Inner Guru

I think ninety-nine times and find nothing. I stop thinking, swim in silence, and the truth comes to me.

Albert Einstein

I am a proud, card-carrying introvert. That doesn't mean I don't like people or parties, it just means that I need time by myself to reconnect with my inner wisdom. My husband is an extrovert. Extroverts need to be around people to recharge. I used to feel that there was something wrong with me because I didn't like to party all the time or be around a lot of friends all the time. Our society can be pretty judgmental. Now I embrace my quiet side. I honor it. It has been in my moments of solitude when I have received the most significant guidance. When things are noisy, when I am focused on what is going on outside of me, I get distracted.

The way most of us lead our lives, moments of solitude are few and far between. For some, the only solitude they have is while sleeping or in the bathroom. The most important relationship we will ever have is with ourselves. Some people might think that as a mother that suggestion is sacrilegious, but it is true. We have enormous responsibility for the well-being of our children, but that does not negate the fact that we are the only ones who never leave us...ever. You were born with you, you breathe every breath with you, and you will die with you. In fact, if you are a parent, allowing your kids to see you valuing yourself enough to carve out sacred solitude teaches them an incredibly important lesson about self-love.

We each have a powerful energy source, Divine Love, within us. Whatever you label it, when you are focused on the minutia of life— on moving from one task to the next, on busyness—you can't feel this energy. It is only in silence, of body and monkey brain, that you feel this energy pulsing…and it really does pulse. It reminds you that you don't need to figure out the next four steps to take to achieve your dreams, because when you listen to this energy source, it tells you your next step, through intuition and signs all around you, precisely when you need to know it. It is God holding you in the palm of His hand. It reminds you that you are perfectly fine in this moment. It reminds you that you are connected by a web of energy to every person, animal, plant, and etheric presence that exists.

Meditation has become important to me. It's like plugging myself into a charger. Many people are intimidated by meditation, and I understand why. It takes practice to quiet the body and the mind. We aren't a patient bunch. Pop culture spirituality, as it has become en vogue, creates ego competition. Can you perform the poses correctly in yoga, and in a room as hot as the Amazon rainforest? Do you cleanse? When you meditate, do you transcend? Here's the truth: we are all spiritual already. You do not need to do anything to become more so. Where I think we could use some help is in connecting to the inner guru within each of us instead of looking to *experts*. For some people, yoga helps. For others, it's nature walks alone, running, or saying the Rosary.

I have personally found that transformation comes for me in the space between my thoughts. Getting silent long enough to have space between my thoughts is something my monkey brain and I have worked a lot on. Spending time by myself, in nature or meditating, is the best way I have found to tap into that. Being perfectly still connects me to the river of wisdom within. It's a mighty river.

Meditation is simply quiet reflection or contemplation. There are many approaches. I don't personally believe you should try to control your thoughts in meditation. Feel free to notice your thoughts as they drift by—just don't attach to them. It is the absence of control that is at the heart of meditation. It's about letting go of our illusion of control. These are the moments when I realize I don't need to do a darn thing to heal myself because there is a greater Source that knows what is best for me. It's not surprising that during a meditation I heard

"I am exactly where I am supposed to be". That's the kind of guidance we ignore when we are racing through life. During my quiet moments I sometimes receive profound ideas about the nature of life. These are the moments when I feel like I am floating on a river, lovingly protected and guided. It's amazing. I have also had to learn that the exercise of being quietly present is a gift itself. Do not go in expecting life-altering insights. The insights ONLY come for me when I am not looking for them, which is a little frustrating when you want to control things which you can't. This makes the regular practice that much more important to establish so you'll be open to it when it wants to pop in and rock your world.

Thomas Edison was fascinated by the ethereal (nonphysical) world around us. One of his last projects before he died was attempting to build a telephone to connect with the dead. Even before working on this device, Edison was known for meditating several times per day to gain inspiration. Edison believed there is a veil between being awake and asleep and in that moment we are most connected to our souls, our higher consciousness. He would sit in a chair holding ball bearings in each loosely closed hand and would set metal pie tins on the floor beneath his hands. As he drifted off, the ball bearings would fall into the pie tins, waking him instantly. He would immediately write down any impressions, sights, or sounds that he was thinking of in that moment. I wonder if that's where the inspiration for the lightbulb came from…

I also have amazing walking meditations in nature. Nature is a chorus of inspiring sounds. This chorus has the power to connect us to the larger web of life. I walk every day at a nature preserve. Sometimes I walk with people, and sometimes I walk alone. Walking alone offers me the chance to connect with my inner wisdom by following the constant drum of nature's own rhythms. Birds and insects sing their own rhythmic songs. My favorite of these is the powerful sounds of the cricket. Sometimes I find myself drifting into a heightened state just by standing in proximity to a cricket hidden in the brush playing me her sweet, organic violin. Even if you live in a city, the white noise can be powerfully soothing if you allow it.

Whatever approach calls to you, please consider spending time in silence connecting to the part of you that already knows her worth and her power, the part of you that will help you to connect with God. It is an art that must be practiced to be mastered so keep at it even when you feel like you'll never "get there".

7.

Your Life Is like a Movie

All the world's a stage, and all the men and women merely players: they have their exits and their entrances; and one man in his time plays many parts, his acts being seven ages.

William Shakespeare

Whether it is a great novel or film, detaching ourselves from our reality and getting lost in a great story is something most of us revel in. As human beings, we love to feel emotions vicariously, even the icky ones, but we don't like the fear and anguish that comes with feeling them in our personal lives. What draws us to fiction is not only enjoying a story, but the possibility of feeling these emotions in a safe setting.

Quantum physicists are theorizing that our world is a projection, a field to play life on. If you have ever seen the movie *The Matrix*, perhaps you have an appreciation for what I mean. I don't believe there are cyborgs feeding off of us, but what if what we say is *real* is just projections from our consciousness made evident by what we choose to focus on? Trippy...

Your life is one great saga. You are the main character. You have a supporting cast, some of whom stay with you for long segments and others that pop in for a particular event and then pop out. The director is your soul. The me that plays me in the movie doesn't know what is coming next, although she would *really* like to. The player doesn't see the plot twists up ahead, but keeping your vibration high seems to help steer the way the plot unfolds. Not knowing the future is part of the magic. Can you imagine how boring your life movie would be if you knew what each day would bring? Not too many people would pay money to experience that.

The challenges that our characters face propel us to new abilities, adventures, and insights. Rocky Balboa had to lose so that he could tap into his inner determination to come back. Ray Kinsella had to almost lose his farm in *Field of Dreams* to prove he had the faith to continue on his mystical journey. Katniss Everdeen had to *volunteer* for the Hunger Games in order to become the beacon of hope for the revolution, and Andy Dufresne had to be falsely convicted of killing his wife and her lover in order to show us that hope never dies in *The Shawshank Redemption*.

I met a beautiful soul, Sue, one morning as I watched the sunrise in Kingston. This woman lost her home to a fire several months earlier. She and her husband lost all of their possessions. When I met her, she was living in a five-hundred-square-foot bungalow near the beach. She told me she had four plates, four utensils, four glasses, etc....and she told me she had never been happier. I am sure she was very unnerved by the fire and the loss, and yet she received a gift that was so much more profound—simplicity—and she *knew* it.

After going through cancer, many people reinvent themselves in a more authentic way. How many wildly successful entrepreneurs endured complete failures (bankruptcy, job loss, even homelessness) before making it big? Is it scary? At first, yes. If you try to hide from challenges, you are hiding from life. How you handle challenges, whether you see opportunities or obstacles, is entirely up to you. If you believe it will destroy you, it just might, but if you ride the wave, chances are it will bring you to better shores.

The movie that is your life will have highs and lows. Learn the lessons from fiction that all heroes and heroines must taste life in the abyss before tasting the ecstasy of triumph. Fully expect that your life will have highs and lows. Sit back and enjoy the show. Don't sweat the abyss. Learn from it. Trust that you won't stay there forever. When it is time to rise up, a ladder will appear.

8.

I am Not Fearless, but I Know How to Use My Fear

The only thing we have to fear is fear itself.

Winston Churchill

We come into this world utterly vulnerable and at the mercy of life, and yet we trust. In early childhood, we hold everything that we encounter in a state of wonder. As we grow through experiences, we begin to believe that we are separate from one another, oh the joy of social conditioning. Some of us begin to believe that we have to work hard to get anything we want and that the world is a scary place of diseases, predators, and lack. Some of us learn to fear life.

Did you sign your child up for the second sport of the season because you were worried he might fall behind the competition, even though it meant he would have no downtime to simply play outside in the afternoon? Did you take more than you needed because you feared they would run out—which probably happened because collectively we fear lack and so many of us take more than we can use? Did you buy a car that was a bit more than you could afford because it suggested an image of success and status that you wanted to project? These are the kinds of things we all do or have done. These decisions are based on false projections that we can label fear.

We have been living in a fear-based world. We feel small and separate. Our media loves to report on any story that will scare the bejeezus out of us. We are addicted to being scared, angry, and disenchanted! We learn to stay in line—to follow, not lead—in order to stay safe. Life isn't always easy. We get dealt some tough hands from time to time, but making fear-based decisions won't make it any easier. In fact, I firmly believe that living from a fear-based perspective, a not-enough, not-safe point of view, simply aligns you with having more fear-based experiences or no experiences at all.

When we live from fear, we try to protect what we possess. It seems to me that if we have to dig our nails into something to prevent it from going, then it wasn't meant for us in the first place or was meant for us for a time that has now passed. Release the death grip! We hold on for dear life to jobs that suck the life out of us, people that make us feel less than we are, homes that no longer fit our needs, and personas and ideas about who we think we are when, in fact, we are just sojourners traveling through these life experiences.

Fear can look like jealousy, anger, and worry. It can look like micro-managing, copying what others do and have, and it can look like depression and an inability to move forward. I am a recovering fear-based liver. It wasn't until I actually got a scary diagnosis that I finally learned to let go of my fear. And that's the kicker, the challenges that we fear so much actually release us from the fear! *Tricky universe...*

Fear has its place, like encouraging us to run faster from that man-eating tiger, but it was not meant to be the basis of our day-to-day decisions. My favorite acronym for fear is **false evidence appearing real**.

It's wise to learn to distinguish between true fear for your safety and false fear 'what ifs'. One problem is that excitement or nervous energy, can feel like fear. It's easy to confuse the feelings. It's important to honor the feeling without letting it control you or your choices. I have learned that I will always be uncomfortable when I try something new. It's just who I am, but knowing that about myself I can now notice the difference between fear of unsupportive choices and worry that I might make an ass of myself. Recognizing that everything I experience is here for my benefit, for my growth, even when it comes in terrifying packaging, means that I am not a slave to fear anymore and that is a fucking miracle!

Conventional oncology had a horrible track record with brain cancer, so rather than cling to hope in a system that would fail me, I opened myself to everything under the sun, with no beliefs or dogma attached to any of it. I said many times, "I have nothing to lose." Having nothing to lose is a powerful place to be.

It brought me to nutrition, people who had healed their own cancers naturally, spirituality, forces that I couldn't see but made their presence known, and more than anything, the understanding that I am not in control, but am the lead character in the story of my life. No amount of striving or pushing could get me where I need to be any faster. The best I can do is to keep myself focused on good vibrations, just like the Beach Boys suggested. I follow the trail of breadcrumbs that Divine Love provides, because Divine Love is with me in every moment. For someone who used to try to control EVERYTHING, figuring out that I don't have to figure it all out brought me immense peace.

Each time you are presented with a choice, feel where the energy is coming from. If you feel tight, constricted, or your heart is racing, ask yourself: what you are worried will happen if you don't do what you are contemplating? Is it reasonable? Learn to appreciate the difference between the discomfort of defending (fear) and the discomfort of growing (love). Ask God to give you a clear sign of which path to take. If you wait for the cues, Divine Love will always show you the way that serves you most.

9.

We Reap What We Sow

Don't judge each day by the harvest you reap, but by the seeds that you plant.

Robert Louis Stevenson

I am an appallingly bad gardener, which is ironic and apropos considering this insight. I never saw the point in fighting for lettuce, tomatoes, or cucumbers against rabbits, deer, dogs, pests, extreme heat, and mold. It's just a whole lot easier to go to the farm stand. When it comes to the gardens that are our bodies and our minds, there is no farm stand. We are the only gardeners available and if we don't tend to it, our garden will wither and die.

A few years ago, I went to a trance healer. This is something I hadn't experienced before, where an intuitive surrenders herself temporarily to allow spiritual guidance to speak directly to clients. In fact, the trance healer, who became a dear friend of mine, does not even remember what is said during the sessions. It is as if she is sent away. This woman knew only my first name, not my health status. At this first meeting, the spiritual entity through the medium told me that "I am the flower." What did that mean?

That happens to me a lot. I go out seeking answers and instead get more questions! This is my pattern because the answers are always within me, not a guru. Good teachers do not give you all the answers, but provide breadcrumbs that lead you within yourself, where your answers are. The first thing I did was buy a potted daisy. I studied it. It revealed nothing to me. It died...from lack of care.

I began to contemplate flowers. A seed starts its life cycle in the dark, damp, cold dirt. The thrust of movement to break open from its shell cannot feel comfortable. Nor can the upward climb to the surface, not knowing what awaits it. An inevitable part of the growth cycle is challenging what we know. We must do this. Once above ground, the stem reaches up and up toward the sun, and below the ground, downward ever further to root itself securely in the earth, until it is finally ready to unfurl itself in glory. The seed must go through this process of growth in order to bloom. *The seed must trust life and how it is unfolding.* Do you see the symmetry?

Just like a flower, I must be patient with the answers I seek. Even if I want something yesterday, there is a divine order running the show that has a better sense of perfect timing than I do. Flowers bloom when nature decides that they are ready to bloom and not one minute before.

Trying to explain God is like trying to explain why water is wet. God is ineffable. It's just beyond description. I have come up with a metaphor for my relationship with God that helps me to feel my connection. I picture God as Mother Earth. I picture people as flowers growing out of God's soil. We are each unique and each intended to bloom at different times. We grow from seeds, break through challenges, grow toward the light, blossom, and then wither and return to Mother Earth to help her grow more flowers.

Just like a garden that you begin working on in April, patience is key. In the spring, you plant the seeds. You must then pull the weeds as they start to grow and also water regularly. Sometimes you need to do some pest control and some fertilizing—*natural, of course.* Eventually you reach harvest time, but only after you have diligently worked through the seasons. Your garden grows on God's timetable, not yours.

We are all flowers in the end, but to bloom, we go through many stages of growth. Flowers don't bloom the day after they are planted. They need just the right nutrients, sunlight, and time. The payout happens later. We reap what we sow.

My body and mind were unruly for a long time. I hadn't tended to them. I spent most of my time trying to distract myself from my untended, overgrown garden. My garden had a lot of weeds growing, got used to pesticides that killed everything, didn't get enough sun or nutrients, and therefore everything was wet and moldy.

When we have a diseased human garden, mental or physical, we shouldn't expect it to bloom overnight. Growth is a sacred process that cannot be rushed. Practice patience and care, and use a good barrier to keep out invaders. Get yourself a pair of good gardening gloves and pull out your seed journal, like the one you used in kindergarten, to track your growth. Marvel at the changes that are occurring within your body and your mind each day. You might enjoy witnessing the growth process so much that you forget about blooming and in doing so, you already have.

10.

Don't Attach to Pain

The aim of the wise is not to secure pleasure, but to avoid pain.

Aristotle

This can so easily become a pattern. It was a powerful crutch for me. When I was diagnosed with a brain tumor, it gave me a bit of a free pass in many people's eyes. I found myself able to say what I thought without quite the backlash I might have expected if I didn't have the diagnosis. I liked that feeling. I liked feeling immune to criticism. I liked being able to talk about alternative cancer treatments, pharmaceutical poisons, and GMOs without being personally attacked as so many others who are trying to bring awareness are. I liked that the brain tumor made me feel special in a sad sort of way. I also liked that if things got too tough I could use the brain tumor as an excuse. I even occasionally used it in arguments with my husband.

Energetically, my body and surroundings started catching on to this self-sabotaging cycle. Just as I would gear up to start my blog, make a big push to get my business thriving, or go after another goal, my health status would conveniently get scary or would *require, I thought,* my undivided attention—or my kids would get lice (true story). It became a pattern. It became my comfort zone. I was so good at getting 90 percent there and then pulling back.

Many people use their pain like a crutch. It becomes the excuse for why they can't change this or that. People get so attached to their ailments that they forget how it feels to be well. By focusing on the challenge, they feed more energy into it, creating more pain to complain about. I know because this was me and I see it in many people. Eventually your pain becomes like superglue if you are always thinking and talking about it. I don't choose to attach myself to the brain tumor any longer. If it's there, it's there (or not), but that doesn't stop me from living in this moment. In fact, how can I not see it as a blessing when so much transformation has resulted from it? I sincerely hope that I am around until I am 90, but if I exit stage right before then, I am comforted in knowing that I woke up from my slumber in time to truly relish in this life. This is the moment we have been given. Use it or lose it.

Do you do this? Are you attached to pain in your life, a *poor me* moment, a victim story that keeps you small, that you run back to when things get too tough and scary? Let it go. Stop clinging. In clinging to a pain crutch, you are preventing yourself from moving forward. There are bound to be scary things up ahead, but why hold on to pain? You know that doesn't feel good. All that it feels is familiar.

11.

I Am the Proverbial Onion

Life is like an onion. You peel it off one layer at a time, and sometimes you weep.

Carl Sandburg

In the last century, we invested a lot of time, money, and effort into creating conveniences. Can you imagine what it would be like to spend one day in 1901? The transformation has been mind blowing. The Internet didn't go mainstream until the mid-1990s. These conveniences have made our lives so comfortable, and yet in our zeal to make our lives easier, we have given control to others to solve our problems when they arise. We often fail to take responsibility time and again for what we experience. This is true of healing, reaching for more fulfilling jobs or even reaching life goals.

When I started this healing journey in 2010, even though I chose the holistic path, I was still looking for someone to fix me. I was searching for the magic bullet. My search turned up a fascinating truth, one I was not that happy to learn. Divine timing has the wheel no matter how my ego might bully it. I had to learn to be patient. I had to learn to be contented with where I was. That's not so bad if life is going along okay, but when you have a crisis, you want answers yesterday!

I could never have predicted in July 2010 where I would be now. My prognosis told me I might be in rough shape by now, if not dead. I had to separate myself from the fear surrounding cancer. I had to learn to let life unfold. I had to learn that the right information would make its way to me if I kept my heart and head clear and if I waited for it to find me. If you have a scary life issue, I know you feel like you are going to snap if you don't figure out the end result, but you can't and you aren't meant to. You are supposed to ride the wave of life, not try to control the ocean.

With time, I began to see the layer upon layer of uncluttering that I am now experiencing. While for the first couple of years I focused on the physical—eating the right foods, taking the right supplements, etc.— as time passed and I gained a broader perspective I found that it was my mind, not my body, that needed my TLC more. While I still eat cleanly most of the time, I try to only do things that align with good mental health. I am okay that the brain tumor didn't disappear with a magic bullet. It would have been nice, but it wasn't my path. I have to be okay with it, it's clearly what I am meant to experience so why fight it? I know two people whose brain cancer healed very quickly on holistic programs. If mine had, I would have missed out on so many insights, so much personal transformation, and so much deep-level healing.

I believe it is how much we can let go of—not how much we can handle—that defines our power. Healing anything is about pulling back the layers of crap that we have coated our lives with. I'll be honest, healing often means two steps up and one step back. Healing is about expressing our authentic selves. Healing is multilayered and is not subject to my timetable. It helped me relax into the flow. Sometimes I cry, as working with onions will do, but the layers are getting far easier to strip, so I know I am getting closer to center. Give yourself the time and space to heal your toxic habits, toxic food, and toxic feelings. Trust the unfolding. It's in Divine order.

12.

Play like Your Life Depends on It

Follow your bliss and the universe will open doors where there were only walls.

Joseph Campbell

Recently I was waiting for an appointment and watched a five-year-old boy, who looked strikingly like me when I was five—*thanks for the Dorothy Hamill haircut Mom*—play with toys. He was fully engrossed in stacking wooden toys inside a toy toolbox. He was fully focused on that one moment. He reminded me of me when I was his age. Watching him was like a meditation for me. I realized how little of this exists for us now. Even our young children rarely play by themselves without rules or electronic sounds. I wasn't surprised to discover that he was Italian, visiting from Italy with his mother. I don't see American children playing like this anymore.

I was incredibly imaginative as a child. In fact, I was in my own little world a lot of the time. Around the age of eight, I determined that to get attention it was best for me to focus on left-brain logical and measurable accomplishments as I would receive more positive attention that way. I let my creativity and my sense of fun and play atrophy.

I became very serious. I approached everything as if it was a challenge rather than an opportunity. Getting the cancer diagnosis just confirmed that life was not child's play. Then I started meeting highly intuitive people. I started receiving messages from the other side. Whether it was angelic guides or my father, I heard repeatedly that I needed to play. Many people would immediately jump at this suggestion. I balked at it. "Play? Who's got time for that? I've got to heal my body! I've got to help people by sharing the truth of holistic healing!" Play would have to wait...

The truth is that I had forgotten how to enjoy my life. I no longer knew how to play or what I actually liked to do. I love to read, to watch movies, and to take nature walks by myself or with my family and my dogs. I also needed to connect with my inner child whom I had unceremoniously kicked to the curb. I have begun borrowing my son's Rollerblades. I have also begun to color again. I'm not painting; I'm coloring in adult coloring books with pencils. It's easy, relaxing, and rewarding. I am also a newbie knitter. I watch my free-spirited, anti-establishment daughter skip, and I feel the desire to skip. Every time I play outside the box, I am exercising my creative brain.

I am logical enough. My left brain needs a break, not a workout. I have learned that enjoying life is paramount to healthy living. It's one of the reasons I have eased up on the strictness of my diet. I want to enjoy life, to live in joy with life. Playing is experiencing. I am here to experience life, not to analyze it.

13.

Messages from the Ethers

Without the spiritual world the material world is a disheartening enigma.

Joseph Joubert

When we are standing near a window and the rays of the sun begin to shine through, we get a glimpse of tiny particles circulating in the air that are otherwise invisible to us. We assume the air is empty space, but it's definitely not. I haven't experienced death, so I can't say exactly what happens after this life, but what I do know is that the other side of the veil, the nonmaterial, invisible world, is ALWAYS communicating with us. I sincerely hope that this knowledge is a source of comfort to all those who have lost a loved one.

From the near-death accounts that I have read and the spiritual communicators that I have met or seen, I can say that I certainly do not believe in a punishing God or a hell beyond that which we create in our own minds. A consistent message from those who have glimpsed the other side is that our loved ones are with us all the time, that Heaven is the state of the nonphysical rather than a place, that time does not exist, so everything that has happened or ever could, happens simultaneously, that we have an immense creative partnership with Divine Love that can help us shape our 'future' through our dominant vibration and that we are indescribably loved exactly as we are.

Earlier I wrote about how my father connected with me at the time of his passing, something two other people I have met also experienced at the time of their loved one's passing. Not being physically present was a common denominator. I also told you of the dream I had the night before my surgery in which my father reassured me that he was still near. I have many other stories as well, including both of my dogs giving us clear signals of their presence after they had passed.

About eighteen months after my father passed away, I went to see a medium in a small group setting at a place of healing called Hope Floats. I was with nineteen other people, many skeptical, including me. The medium, a young twentysomething woman, brought through the first loved one, who she was able to say died in Afghanistan in a rollover accident. She even displayed his signature joke. When it was my turn, she said to me, "Your dad walked in here with you tonight." I hadn't told her I was there to connect with my father. She then said, "Your father is helping you now more than he could before," which made me begin to sob. You see, my dad was a very straight-laced guy. He would never have supported my alternative approach to healing. In fact, he may have been very *unsupportive.* I had been telling people for the previous eighteen months that I had a sense that my father was guiding me to the right steps and that he was helping me more now than he could have before. The medium told me exactly what I had been telling others. There were several other amazing insights, like her knowing about the cancer and about a conversation I had with only my husband six months earlier about getting a product I was supporting into Whole Foods. My father said through the medium that "whatever I could imagine I could achieve."

I believe that we receive continual messages from the divine in order to guide us along our life path. Throughout 2012, I kept hearing the name *John of God.* John of God is a powerful unconscious medium who lives in rural Brazil. John of God considers himself an instrument in God's divine hands. According to his website, he does not claim to cure anybody, but rather, he gives over his consciousness to the spirits of past doctors and saints to heal and console us. It is estimated that he has treated, either directly or indirectly, up to fifteen million people during the past forty years. I am one of them.

One of my favorite spiritual teachers, Wayne Dyer, credits John of God with healing him of leukemia. Wayne Dyer passed away from heart failure on August 30, 2015. After his John of God experience, he chose to no longer be tested for leukemia markers, something I have chosen as well. The problem that many people have with this decision is like what the skeptics will say: "You have no proof you are healed." I have had to learn to accept that, because the stress of the testing does far more damage to me than ignoring naysayers. According to the coroner's report, Wayne Dyer had no trace of leukemia in his body, confirming his claim of healing with John of God. I also read the amazing testimony of a man with glioblastoma multiforme, the most aggressive type of brain tumor, who fully healed after living at John of God's Casa retreat for a few years. His story can be found in the New York Times bestseller *Radical Remission: Surviving Cancer against All Odds*, [5] which shares nine key factors in healing "incurable" cancers. Pretty fascinating and *out there* stuff, right?

Oprah Winfrey has interviewed John of God at the Casa de Dom Inácio de Loyola, named for Saint Ignatius Loyola—one of the regular entities that comes to heal and the founder of the Jesuit order of Catholic priests—where John of God resides and conducts his work. John of God also does not accept payment for his services.

I know that when I hear the same name, or supplement, or exercise, etc., from multiple sources that it is a message. That is what happened for me with John of God. Although a trip to Brazil would have been fascinating, it was not likely to happen. In January 2013, after yet another prompting of the name John of God, I began to research him again. This time I discovered that he had a distance healing option in which dedicated guides present your picture along with healing requests to him. The cost is approximately seventy dollars, which covers the cost of energy-enhanced supplements fitted to your exact energetic healing needs and the cost of shipping them to the United States. The passionflower supplements come with instructions to take them for about fifty days and to avoid spicy foods and alcohol in that time. All this sounds nuts, I know, but just hold on…

My guide, a woman from the UK, e-mailed me to let me know my picture would be presented to John of God on that coming Thursday around 1:00 p.m. My healing requests were for healing of the brain tumor, naturally, as well as for financial support. Healing naturally is not cheap, mainly because my insurance will not cover vitamins, energy work, body work, or my nutritionist, and that's all I do. If you could see me, you would know that I am very healthy right now whether a tumor is still present or not. In fact, I am far healthier than I was prior to my diagnosis.

My guide told me that I could meditate during this time, but didn't have to. I wasn't that adept at meditation then, but I did quiet myself at 1:00 p.m. for about thirty minutes and I felt...*NOTHING.* She told me that she would e-mail me a few days later if I required psychic surgery or with any special instructions.

That night while I was sleeping, I had the most vivid dream of my life. There was a man in my dream whom I had never laid eyes on before. Now, that alone is really odd as I can't recall ever having a dream about a stranger. This man kept smiling at me. He totally freaked me out. He didn't threaten me in any way, but everywhere I turned I found him directly in front of me, smiling. He had brown bouffant hair and piercing brown eyes. When I awoke Friday morning, I shared my dream with my husband, Mike. I told him how freaky the whole thing was. It didn't even cross my mind that this could be connected to John of God. Over the next three days, I couldn't get this man from my dreams out of my mind.

On Sunday evening, three days later, I heard back from my guide. She told me I had no special instructions other than to take the passionflower supplements as directed until they were gone. The package would arrive in about three weeks—the Casa is in rural Brazil. She told me that the entity who came through John of God for my healing was Dr. Augusto de Almeida, a Casa "regular." I was curious to find out any information I could about this spirit doctor, so I Googled him. My husband was standing next to me as I typed in his name, witnessing my stunned reaction when his image (a painting) revealed that Dr. Augusto de Almeida was my mystery dream man. I KID YOU NOT. That man who showed up in my dream the night of my healing was in fact my healer! I am 100 percent certain of it. I started yelling excitedly to my husband, "That's the guy, that's the guy from my dream!"

I began taking my passionflower supplements when they arrived. After about three weeks, I began to realize that my fear of the brain tumor was gone! Fear (or stress) prevents healing. Up until this point, I had done my best to live my life one moment at a time, but I always carried this heavy, fearful energy below the surface. Like magic, I realized that I had no fear. Although the brain tumor was still present on MRIs after that, the fear was gone. Matter (e.g., the brain tumor) is slower vibrating energy, so healing myself on the energetic level (a faster energy) will precede the physical.

With only about a week left of supplements, I received the answered healing for my other request as well, in a very unlikely way. On the Saturday night before Easter, my daughter Kyra said she smelled gasoline. I immediately went down to our basement. When I opened the door, our storage area, where our furnace is, was engulfed in heavy black smoke. I ran up the stairs yelling for everybody to get out of the house. We called the fire department right away and made a huge spectacle of ourselves, as you might imagine. The fire department determined it was a furnace malfunction. We had a lot of smoke damage and lost a lot of what we had stored there. I even lost all the Easter candy and gifts for the following morning and found myself scouring Dick's, Old Navy, Michaels, and Target at 8:50 p.m. for replacements.

Now although this sounds like anything but the answer to my prayers, it was, in fact, a huge blessing. Not only did we get rid of a lot of stuff that was just taking up space, but we also received a very good insurance settlement to cover our lost possessions, and we had our house cleaned, top to bottom, by a professional restoration crew that became my housemates for a week.

So beyond these two amazing outcomes, what else did I learn? I learned through this experience that I don't always (or even often) know what is best for me or how it should arrive. When I surrendered myself, when I turned myself over to God, I opened myself to what God wanted for me at that moment. It was the beginning of a rapid spiritual awakening. It made me know that I am watched over, loved, and protected in all that I do. The experience instilled patience in me. There are no accidents.

Trust in the process of life and trust in Divine Love. You can ride this roller coaster holding onto the bar for dear life or with your hands up over your head. The choice is yours.

14.

Focusing On Your Problems Amplifies Them

Where attention goes energy flows.

James Redfield

Have you ever heard that we teach what we need to learn? Well, that's me, and this particular lesson is still a work in progress. I don't blame myself for being slow to learn it. In fact, I never blame myself or anyone else for anything anymore. I am really proud that I am where I am with it because many people never get close. If you focus on your problems, you are energetically feeding those problems and drawing more similar experiences to you. This does not contradict accepting where you are. Accepting yourself as you are is a primary condition of self-love. It is your starting point, but dwelling on what isn't working is when we get on the hamster wheel to nowhere.

I always focused on the problems in my life. Truly I did. If there was a glass to be seen, to me, it was always half-empty. And then God gave me the ultimate tool to learn this most critical lesson. I was given a brain tumor with God challenging me to find the gift in it. Had it been anything smaller, I would have bitched and moaned and thought, "Why me?" I would have done things by the book, whatever the book said to do, and I would have continued on in a small, closed-in life or died. For me to learn, it had to be a colossal challenge.

I am an equal-opportunity challenger to the status quo, so rather than talk about the evils of Monsanto, I am going to challenge the well-intentioned people working hard to make changes to our food and medicine supply and to those focused on saving the planet. First, I used to be one of them. I completely admire them for what they are trying to do, but I feel that sometimes they are going about it wrong, energetically speaking. When you are focused on flaws, on what is wrong, on finger-pointing, you are feeding angry, powerful energy to that very problem and you are looking for enemies!

In my personal healing journey, I was always looking for another supplement, practice, or process to heal me. Every time I did, I was feeding energy to "I'm not healed." When I looked at pharmaceutical companies and agro-conglomerates and thought, "This is what is wrong with the world," I fed momentum into the very system I was hoping to change. Change is happening. It's undeniable, but it feels like when the agents of change focus on what is desired, such as people choosing natural food, we change faster, but when we focus on what Monsanto does wrong, we get stuck in the mud. One of the most inspirational figures in history, Dr. Martin Luther King Jr., said in his most famous "I have a dream" speech that "there is something that I must say to my people, who stand on the warm threshold which leads into the palace of justice: In the process of gaining our rightful place, we must not be guilty of wrongful deeds. Let us not seek to satisfy our thirst for freedom by drinking from the cup of bitterness and hatred. We must forever conduct our struggle on the high plane of dignity and discipline. We must not allow our creative protest to degenerate into physical violence. Again and again, we must rise to the majestic heights of meeting physical force with soul force." Dr. King knew it. You cannot change anything from the same consciousness that created it. Hate will never drive hate from our hearts. Dare to envision your reality the way you want it and keep your mind on that greater state, not on what's terrible about today.

We can also learn some valuable lessons from people in our own lives who seem completely disengaged from making the world a better place. These are people who spend all their time in their own worlds, not in the global arena. They don't watch the news. They don't read anything depressing. They live in a highly controlled world of their design, and they do not let negativity pollute what they have created. These people seem untouched and unconcerned by most of society's problems. They rarely rally against corporations and never post controversial topics on Facebook. They have great vacations, perfectly coiffed children, and expectations of success in everything they do. Usually they get what they want, too.

Some readers might already be feeling resentful about these people, but you know what? *They figured it out.* They figured out how to get what they want by focusing *only* on what they want and not entertaining what they don't. I think many of these people have an easier time attracting their hearts' desires because these people often want what society says is most desirable, like material wealth, so they do not have internal conflict, but these people are not the enemy. They are just living their lives. If the change agents were able to put aside judging the lifestyle many of these people chose, they could learn a lot about how to create the world they want.

I watched an amazing YouTube video that Gregg Braden shared from a medicine-less hospital in China where tumors evaporate through the power of focused intention in which energy practitioners chant the equivalent to "already healed." Gregg Braden was a computer geologist for Phillips Petroleum, a senior computer systems designer with Martin Marietta Defense Systems, and the first technical operations manager for Cisco Systems, clearly a qualified and respected scientist. He is also renowned for bridging science and spirituality. In the three-minute video, you can actually watch a kidney tumor disappear on an ultrasound. The patient wasn't even a part of the chanting or belief and yet she healed because of the depth of belief the energy healers had that the woman was "already healed." I hope you'll look it up.

I work with a highly intuitive chiropractor. She is very much the traditional medicine woman without much medicine, except occasional turmeric and fish oil. She always knows where my thoughts and feelings are. One day not long ago, I was working on writing a version of this book that I scrapped because of its more frustrated, negative tone. I had cleared myself of a lot of the feeling of "being sick" in the previous year, but writing the book was feeling heavy, like I was dredging up the muck from the bottom of a marsh. I was writing a lot about having a brain tumor and was beginning to think about it from a place of fear and anger again.

My chiropractor, who was unaware of my writing and had told me at several previous appointments that my head felt very clear, all of a sudden handed me the prayer card of St. Peregrine, the patron saint of cancer patients. She then said to me, "Focus on what you want, not on what you don't." She had nailed it. Even though writing about this experience is something I was meant to do and is part of the gift of the tumor, by going at it from a place of frustration and anger I had temporarily reactivated the physical energy of the tumor. After the appointment, I committed myself to writing everything from a place of acceptance, not fear (or anger and resentment). At the very next appointment, only a week later, without me telling her anything about my writing, she said things felt clear again.

This brings me to a tool that has been so trivialized by our society that we relegate it only to children: imagination. Our imagination can create any reality we want. Rather than focusing on what I don't want—my former pattern of choice—I now focus on only what I do want. I can imagine my body in beautiful health. I can imagine a world where the oceans are clean, food is healing, and people have plenty and are happy rather than stressed. I can even imagine that Monsanto is making products that benefit humanity. It's not that I am being obtuse. It's not that I am being naïve. I am exercising my powerful mind to create the reality that I wish to see in the physical world rather than using my mental energy to fight a reality that I don't want.

My neighbor taught me a very valuable lesson a couple years ago about the power of intentional thinking. After going through some difficult life events, he was diagnosed with prostate cancer. Life trauma often precedes cancer. He had biopsies at Massachusetts General Hospital and South Shore Hospital to confirm the presence of cancer. He was not interested in the conventional treatments, nor was he interested in changing his diet with a natural cancer approach. Instead, he forged his own path. He began a daily process of what he termed "positive self-talk." He focused on what he wanted, not on what he didn't, and he HEALED! Doctors could find no evidence of disease. He accomplished this by changing his mind. I believe that virtual reality simulation should be an integral part of our standard of care for all disease so that every patient gets a chance to experience vibrant health.

Don't ignore your challenges, but try seeing them as signs from your soul nudging you to choose differently.

Don't take my word for it. Go out and live it. Stop complaining. Stop judging. Stop attacking your "opposition." Whenever you get upset about the state of something, turn within and imagine it the way you want it. Keep that projection close to you until the material catches up with the ethereal and ignore anyone who tries to burst your bubble. Walk through life with rose-colored glasses and you will be doing more for humanity than your complaining and finger-pointing will ever do.

15.

Stop Proving Your Worth

Wanting to be liked means being a supporting character in your own life, using the cues of the actors around you to determine your next line rather than your own script. It means that your self-worth will always be tied to what someone else thinks about you, forever out of your control.

Jessica Valenti

When babies are born they can't do anything for themselves. They can't eat, walk, talk, or even use the bathroom. They are helpless. We must do everything for them. Yet we love them. We adore them. We make silly faces just to encourage them to coo. They are useless to the planet in traditional terms and yet we honor them as being one of the best things about living. They are authentic. In an artificial world, a taste of authenticity reminds us of our spiritual home.

When that baby starts to grow we start piling on expectations. At first, it's expecting the child to follow our guidance, to not color on the walls or not run into the road. As they grow we expect children to perform well in school. If they dare act out or fail to thrive in the life-sucking reality that school has become we label them. If they fail to go to a four year college we assume they won't amount to anything. So to summarize, we love them for the innocent souls that they are as infants and then we forget all of that and force them to conform to society's interpretation of worthiness.

I used to be so impressed by credentials. I was intimidated by anyone I perceived as smarter, wealthier or more accomplished. I failed to see their soul worth as I was always focused on their material worth. So stupid. My worth is not tied to my income, my state of health, the number of friends I have on Facebook or whether you think I am a good writer. My worth was imprinted on my soul long before I became this human being by God. Maybe we recognize that when we see a baby. We long to feel that way about ourselves as adults, but feel too guilty, as if we aren't worthy. The way I see it, if God allowed us to get this far (to be born) it was no accident. Loving ourselves for simply being present here is God's desire yet many of us choose to live our lives according to man's sense of worthiness rather than the laws of the universe, which is not only ludicrous, but utterly ineffective.

We have been raised to respect degrees. The more letters behind someone's name the more we listen to their opinions, the more worthy we make them, even when our common sense steers us differently. You can certainly go through this life and achieve grand accomplishments. You can build a company, you can build a fortune, you can add a lot of letters to the end of your name, but it won't change your worthiness as a human being. It might make your ego feel better, but the ego would rather hang your hat on your past accomplishments. It's easy to love ourselves when our abs are tight, our bank account is fat and people admire us, but that's not true love. True love is recognizing that your birth is all the credential you will ever need to deserve a great life.

Here's a reality check: you just aren't that special. Neither am I. And that is liberating! Stop trying to prove yourself worthy of anything. Stop living in fear of what other people think. The worthiness you are focused upon is a manmade distinction that on the cosmic scale is meaningless. I remember a scene in *Schindler's List* when the Warsaw Jews were forced into the ghetto. The wealthy Jewish families soon found themselves sharing a single tenement apartment with poor Jewish families. Their education, social stature and even their expensive possessions were stripped from them. At any moment you could lose every possession that you hold dear. What can never be taken from you is your divinely-given worth no matter what your surroundings look like.

I was raised in Christianity. All that it takes to appreciate how ass backward we have it is to spend just a short time studying the work of Jesus Christ, who I truly believe came here as an enlightened being to show us how to live in love. Jesus did not choose authority figures as his disciples. He chose the disenfranchised. He engaged with members of society that the rest of society deemed beneath them. He demonstrated that how we treated the *lowliest* of us was how we treated God because we are ALL part of God.

Even if no one ever appreciates your unique self, in the eyes of God you are worthy. Once you no longer give a damn whether people like or respect you, you will be free in your heart and your mind. When you feel free, you radiate that out. Others will want what you're having. It will have a cascading effect. People will stop caring about the Kardashians and start caring about the passions that burn inside of us.

When we stop proving our worthiness, and honor that we are all worthy, we stop craving external man-made symbols of worth. There is nothing wrong with prosperity, in fact, I see it as a very positive thing. All of us deserve it, but it is not the mark of soul worthiness and is often something we fill ourselves with to mask a barrenness that exists deep within us, a place where our soul longings quietly wait to be welcomed. I recently read a statement, that no matter how big your house, your bank account or how luxurious your car, at the end of your life, your coffin is the same size as that of the homeless man. I think it's wonderful to want material comfort. Who wouldn't rather sleep on a soft bed rather than a cardboard box? But if you place too much emphasis on material gain, you might be missing the bigger picture. You are worthy simply because you exist.

16.

Love the Ordinary

Appreciation of life itself, becoming suddenly aware of the miracle of being alive, on this planet, can turn what we call ordinary life into a miracle.

Dan Wakefield

"Life is not measured by the amount of breaths we take, but by the moments that take our breath away." That sounds lovely and inspiring, and I couldn't disagree more. We all have those amazing moments in life that we can never forget. The births of my children are the two happiest moments of my life, as I'm sure many of you would agree. The euphoria I felt in the car on the way to my father's deathbed, which I discovered was the moment he passed to the other side, will also always be extraordinarily important to me, but we do not build a life on breathtaking moments—we build a life on daily life and that should be beautiful, too.

As I walked this morning with a friend, he mentioned to me that almost all the people he knew hated their jobs. Well, THAT sucks. It is nearly impossible to appreciate the goodness of your life when you are miserable for a large portion of it. It's why most of society looks forward to vacations, that one or two weeks a year when you get a taste of what life would be like if you were spending it doing what you enjoy.

I think my degree in life education, with a master's in scary illness, provided me with a much needed smack in my perspective. In many ways, I am blessed with the gift of broader perspective. I also acknowledge how nice it would be to just be like everyone else, but that is not my journey right now. I understand exactly what those on their deathbeds say about their deep regrets because I was given that same gift, just much earlier when I still had time to make changes so that I did not live with regret. I've seen many versions of the regrets of the dying. *The Huffington Post* published another list of them recently.

At the end of their lives people say:

1. I wish I'd had the courage to live a life true to myself, not the life others expected of me.
2. I wish I hadn't worked so hard.
3. I wish I'd had the courage to express my feelings.
4. I wish I had stayed in touch with my friends.
5. I wish that I had let myself be happier.

Not one of these asks for more breathtaking moments. Not one of these is regret about not going after the brass ring. All are about recognizing the gift of the present moment, of the tapestry of life that is woven together with a stream of everyday events.

I am bored with chasing ecstatic, Facebook-worthy moments. It isn't sustainable, and it is the task of those trying to project happiness rather than truly being happy. If you can't enjoy it without sharing it on Facebook, then it might be approval and attention you seek. If that's the case, take a social media hiatus and get in touch with who you would be if no one was watching.

I have discovered profound joy in the spaces in between—the quiet (and sometimes loud if you have kids) breath of daily life with its inhales and exhales. Here are some of my favorite spaces in between:

1. I enjoy driving to pick up my son after school as I notice my town out the window, listen to the radio, and on the trip home, hear him talk about his day…something that doesn't always come willingly from a thirteen-year-old.

2. I adore my daily walks at Bay Farm and my amazing family there. These nature- and dog-loving peeps fill me with JOY. Nobody cares what kind of car you are driving, nobody cares about your age. I have friends in their twenties and friends in their seventies and I love them

all and their canine companions. It is a place of loving acceptance sans makeup and pretense.

3. I enjoy waking up before 6:00 a.m. and getting organized for the day. I love my morning smoothie, my bone broth, and my cups of tea.

4. My heart skips a beat when my daughter gets off the bus. This glorious, free-spirited ten-year-old usually has her backpack half-opened, contents spilling out of it, and is either happy to be home or scowling about school or bus drama…it happens.

5. I love the honor of teaching my children to navigate our ultracompetitive society while not succumbing to it and maintaining their sense of themselves.

6. I love when dinner is over and my husband, my kids, and I sit down to watch *The Amazing Race*, *Master Chef*, or *Modern Family*.

Life is measured by breath. Some breaths are glorious, some breaths suck, and many leave no traceable emotion. All of it is the breath of life and all of it is glorious if you actually stop to appreciate it.

Ponder your life. Do you love it, hate it, have no opinion about it? Don't wait too long before you figure out what truly matters to you and do everything you can to align yourself with what your heart wants.

A friend shared this quote from Martha Beck, and I just needed to include it here in closing.

> *Our culture has come to define happiness as an experience that blows your mind. It's as though we're somehow falling short if we don't routinely feel the way Times Square looks—madly pulsing with a billion watts of Wow! Don't get me wrong. Excitement is a great and necessary thing; without it life wouldn't be complete. But happiness—real happiness—is something entirely different, at once calmer and more rewarding. And cultivating it is one of the most important steps we can take toward creating fulfilling lives.*

Be real, be honest, and be in love with the gift of everyday, ordinary life.

17.

<u>Soften, Don't Harden to Life</u>

If we can soften our hearts and we can access the pure and simple aspect of our nature, then we can regain the realization that everything we need is already inside us and anything is attainable.

Yehuda Berg

As challenges present themselves in our lives, we often react by stiffening. We stiffen our bodies, we stiffen our resolve, we hold our breath, we get rigid. Hardening isn't good for our arteries, our joints, or our souls. Hardening is actually the worst thing you can do in a car accident. More whiplash results when the driver knows the collision is about to occur and stiffens. When blindsided, if the body is still relaxed, you might not walk away injury-free, but odds are better than if you saw it coming.

When we harden, we are cutting off the flow. Wisdom comes to us most easily when we are in the flow, the flow of the river of life. We grew in the water of our mothers' wombs. We need water to live. Humans can go far longer without food than without water. Water keeps us soft.

I know historically that fear of failure caused me to harden. When I couldn't complete the backward somersault on the balance beam at age eight and was humiliated, I decided that trying new things was scary. When I wasn't sure I could get into Tufts University, I chose not to apply rather than face rejection. When I didn't know what job to take after college (when there weren't a lot of jobs available), I settled for a life-sucking corporate job in a cubicle in financial services for safety.

If you have ever worked with a chiropractor, you know there is pain involved. My chiropractor calls it *pain with a purpose*. I have noticed that I tense up when she starts to work on me. There is a process of building the pocket of energy she is about to dislodge. When the pain starts, my reaction is to stiffen and to hold my breath. As a great chiropractor, she stays with me and keeps pushing me until I finally soften into surrender and breathe into it. Is it easy to soften like that? No, but it isn't something we can avoid, so rather than gingerly peeling a Band-Aid off a hairy arm in slow agony, soften into the pain and just rip that sucker off.

The truth is that the challenges are here to nudge us back into the flow of the river. Too many of us instead stiffen up and back away from the water's edge. It's not always an easy journey on the river of life. We are meant to become like the water. We allow. The river IS life. If we keep hardening with every new challenge, we get brittle. We all know people who live like this. You don't have to. Trust that the flow of life's water is meant to keep you soft and pliable so that you may be carried to the experiences intended for you.

18.

The Pursuit of Happiness Was Making Me Unhappy

Life is a promise; fulfill it.

Mother Teresa

The Founding Fathers of the United States had an enlightened sense of what a great society could be. The fact that the *pursuit of happiness* was a primary message of the Declaration of Independence is extraordinary. But is it happiness or fulfillment that is worth the pursuit?

Ever since I got on this wild ride, I have been pursuing happiness. I heard about it all the time. "Find happiness in everyday circumstances." "Happiness is an inside job." We all know people in our lives that exude happiness.

So what the heck was wrong with me? Why couldn't I be happy? I had done so much soul-searching on this topic. I made it a job! I had gone back in the annals of my mind from early childhood and discovered a truth: happiness is not my driver. Sure, I have had many happy moments, but happiness as an emotion is not the ever-present undercurrent of my life. When you realize something like that—coupled with the awareness that most people use it as a benchmark of a life well lived—you, um, don't feel that great about yourself.

Happiness is a sometimes elusive feeling when you don't know what vehicle to use to get there. Happiness is one emotion in a sea of many that we all experience from time to time. How can I be happy every day? Happiness is, to at least some degree, dependent upon what shows up for you to witness each particular day. If you wake up on a Wednesday and your child is sick, are you really happy or do you feel sad that she doesn't feel well? When someone rear-ends your car, are you happy? Is it realistic to expect that you will be happy then? When the cable company promises they will be at your house between nine and twelve and you wait around and they don't show, are you happy?

I have abandoned my pursuit of happiness and instead have anchored into myself the pursuit of fulfillment. When I follow what calls to me each and every day, I feel fulfilled. When I am of service to others, be it my kids, my husband, a friend, or a stranger, when I write, when I help someone who is in emotional turmoil, I have my best days. Service is profoundly rewarding. It replaces the chasing feeling, the *I am not enough, I don't have enough, I must acquire more* mentality, with *how can I give more?* As I give, I receive. In pursuing fulfillment, I see opportunities. A life of purpose amplifies my opportunities to be happy.

Recently, protesters in Boston blocked two main commuter arteries into the city during rush hour. My husband was caught in one of them and was, thus, late for work. Luckily, he has learned to go with the flow and used the time to meditate. The backlash from the public was swift and harsh. One thing I noticed, though, was that many people mentioned a similar complaint: "It's bad enough that I have to commute to a job I'd rather not go to, now I can't even get there on time!" While I sympathize completely, it made me wonder if these protesters didn't inadvertently stir up emotions of lack of fulfillment in many. I know that wasn't their intention, and I don't agree with their method; I just noticed this sentiment in so much of the angry commentary swirling around. It makes me sad to see people spending so much time at jobs that don't fulfill them. Life is precious—I learned that one the hard way. Life is also far shorter than most of us appreciate. Is it wise to be expending so much energy pursuing something that brings us no fulfillment?

What aspects of your life fulfill you? What aspects deplete you? I have learned to follow whatever lights me up inside. Pursue whatever energizes you...with abandon. This doesn't mean you have to quit your job. I know that isn't realistic—however, be open to opportunities to fulfill your desires. Ask God to bring you opportunities to magnify your purpose. Amazingly, just by answering the questions above, you will have sent a clear signal to God of what you want more of and God will respond with situations to showcase your true colors. The more time you spend in activities that fulfill you, the more likely it is that happiness will come as a result without you having to *pursue* it.

19.

Breaking Out of My Ego's Box of Fear

If you are going through hell, keep going.

Winston Churchill

Surprising as this might sound, I am filled with gratitude and awe when I think of that summer of 2010, and particularly the two-week period from late June through mid-July. During that period in 2010, I juggled the need to be with my dad in Albany, New York, with being in the Boston area getting multiple MRIs, blood work, and the dreaded spinal tap. I let my sisters in on my issue to help cover my tracks, but kept my mother in the dark because I wanted her to focus on my father. I can best describe my mood as *dazed*. It truly felt as though life would never be good again. Not only did I feel like I was losing my rock, but it seemed as though my kids and my husband would be moving on without me. In the words of my oncologist, it was *pretty shitty*.

A few years ago, I became familiar with the term *the Dark Night of the Soul*, which is a vehicle for rapid spiritual awakening. We all live in a box of our ego's construct. We grow up, get a job, find a partner, have children, build a life, and typically never experience anything beyond our self-created world. If we are happy in the world we create, it's pretty good, but if we aren't happy, if we feel unfulfilled in an area of our life, most of us still can't see a way out of the box. We assume that the box keeps us safe even if we aren't very happy in it. We will fight to keep the box together even if it keeps us unfulfilled because it is all we know and we fear the unknown.

The truth, as I see it, is that we are never truly safe until we are our authentic selves. Our souls will not allow us to have our lives dictated by the ego's fear indefinitely because we are all here to experience life in a highly personal way. Most ego boxes are built out of cardboard.

They look tough, but with enough water from the river of life they disintegrate. Our souls are far more powerful than our egos and at any moment can kick the ego's ass. *Firsthand experience with an ass-kicking right here.*

Many souls ultimately *choose* to experience a complete collapse of their ego's box. The more rigid the box we create, the more necessary it is to have a major upheaval manifest to tear it all down. This isn't about God messing with us, but rather a powerful vehicle of transformation. When everything that we have built our lives around comes crashing down, we are allowed to rebuild in a way that is truly authentic to us. Crashing down could mean the loss of a job that wasn't right, disease that ensures life will not go on as usual, the loss of a loved one, a nervous breakdown, or the end of a dysfunctional relationship that we just couldn't seem to leave on our own. These events occur to propel us to immense personal growth and empowerment. The transformation that we undergo during a Dark Night of the Soul changes the way our daily life functions. We can't stop it and there's no use fighting it. What happens next is miraculous if we can muster the courage to surrender to it. When we surrender to it, we begin to know our power and consciousness on a deeper level. That knowing propels us to transform everything else in our lives. Eckhart Tolle has described the Dark Night of the Soul as bringing us to this state:

> *You are meant to arrive at a place of conceptual meaninglessness. Or one could say a state of ignorance—where things lose the meaning that you had given them, which was all conditioned and cultural and so on. Then you can look upon the world without imposing a mind-made framework of meaning. It looks of course as if you no longer understand anything. That's why it's so scary when it happens to you, instead of you actually consciously embracing it.*

In my darkest hour, my self-imposed box that I thought protected me was washed away by the river of life. I was left raw and homeless to pick up the pieces. I honor that time as the most significant of my life. I am so grateful for the moments of God's grace that I experienced after, grace showering down upon me to begin to soothe my raw wounds and to help me find my footing in this brand-new world. Each day I remember another aspect of myself, my true self, and strip away all the crap I had accumulated over a lifetime. Not all of us will experience the Dark Night of the Soul, but many do. Perhaps as a result of reading this, if it happens to you, you won't feel quite so lost. Perhaps you will be able to trust that it will bring blessings and surrender to it.

20.

Seek Information, Not Affirmation

If you don't design your own life plan, chances are you'll fall into someone else's plan. And guess what they have planned for you? Not much.

Jim Rohn

Information is defined as facts provided or learned about something or someone. Affirmation is the confirmation of a truth or validity of a prior judgment. How many times when you believe you are getting information are you actually getting an affirmation for something you already believe? How open are you to a totally new viewpoint? How open are you to shifting your paradigm?

Dogma and our staunch belief that what we have been conditioned to believe is THE right way only serves to keep us from growing and expanding. Dogma is a principle or set of principles laid down by an authority as incontrovertibly true. It serves as the primary basis of an ideology, nationalism, or belief system, and it cannot be changed or discarded without affecting the very system's paradigm. Dogma establishes rules. Rules are designed to control circumstances. Truth is not about control. Truth sets us free. Oppressive regimes have always used control of the flow of information to keep people in line. China censors the Internet. Both Syria and Turkey have recently suspended Internet access as well. Information is never a threat except to those who seek to control others.

Consensus is a powerful force, but one that isn't always to our benefit. Bloodletting was commonplace in medical treatments until the 1800s. In the 1830s, France imported forty million leeches for medical use. I don't think it will be long before conventional wisdom changes its tune on chemotherapy. I look forward to that day. Just because it is conventional wisdom doesn't mean it is right; it only means enough people have come to accept this dogma as true.

Any scientist should be willing to admit that what was believed as fact one hundred years ago is radically different from now, and therefore, what is believed now as fact is only what is believed to be true for this moment in time. Nothing more and nothing less. This can be very difficult for scientists who build careers around one model, system, or belief. Science, as interested as it is in discovering truth, is very hard on hypotheses that challenge conventional scientific theory because the ego fears becoming obsolete.

I have believed many different things in my life. Some of them I continue to believe and some I have long since dismissed, but I strive to be an open vessel, a sponge, waiting for the opportunity for new information to come my way, to test it with my intuition. When I am open, when I am willing to set aside any rigidity with which I believe something, I gain profound insights. I receive powerful intuitive messages now that I follow because if I don't, God has a way of continually bringing the same scenario around again until I finally do pay attention.

The lessons of our parents, teachers, priests, medical professionals, and coaches certainly shape us, but they don't have to define us. There is room for more than one viewpoint. I was raised Catholic. In fact, my father served as parish council president for several years and was a lay minister. My mother was a Eucharistic minister. I went to church every week growing up—although begrudgingly. In high school I attended the teen mass, although I often went to the local ice cream shop instead. Although I went to a Jesuit college, I only went to church maybe six times while I was there, usually for special occasions. I never saw this as making me deficient because I felt that organized religion had too many rules. Being gay was a sin, eating meat on Friday was a sin, not attending mass was a sin. All organized religions have established similar rules that, if followed, lead to salvation. Yet we often forget that many of the most brutal conflicts in human history are a direct result of one group's belief that its way was right and the other's was wrong.

Political views are the same. We align ourselves, usually dependent on our socioeconomic status and geography, to political ideologies. We are right. They are wrong. The Democrats want to destroy the free market economy. The Republicans don't care about the plight of the poor. The same is true for health care. There are two very clear camps: conventional and holistic. Conventional care focuses on pharmaceutical drugs and technological advances, treating the body like car parts, while holistic care focuses on nature and treating the whole being. I think there is benefit to both. As much as I prefer holistic healthcare for healing disease, I want the state of the art trauma center if I am in a car accident.

We are galloping through life like race horses with blinders on. We see what separates us from one another much more than what unites us. Can you imagine as a six-year-old that you are given a set of tenets to follow that will be your truths for the rest of your life with no expansion? As a six-year-old, I thought summertime activities like catching caterpillars and frogs and playing Super Friends (I was the only girl in a boys' neighborhood, so I got to be Wonder Woman) was just about the pinnacle of existence, and at that time it really was! But that clearly wasn't everything, *or maybe life as Wonder Woman would have been awesome!*

Life is change. In our desire to make sense of it all, we reach a point in adulthood where many of us turn off the valve of learning and declare, *I'm full.* We spend the rest of our lives justifying our beliefs. We do this by deciding which media outlet is accurate, which messages and causes we will support, and even which friends we choose to be with.

I am blessed that my husband Mike and I often have deep conversations on the greater meaning of life. We are both on journeys of self-discovery and growth, and we find that God brings us opportunities to engage with, listen to, and learn from each other and, really, everyone and every encounter we have day in and day out. Mike's favorite radio show is a sports show called The Herd with Colin Cowherd. Often he has me listen to a part of the podcasts. I have virtually zero interest in sports other than to find a way to connect with Mike and my son, but I must admit that Colin Cowherd is a very insightful guy. On one show, he was discussing the fact that to be on the radio you pretty much need to choose an extreme. You can be a bleeding-heart liberal, a staunch conservative, a shock jock, or a sports guy. We don't really leave any room in the middle for discussing topics without an agenda.

We often wait in a conversation for our turn to talk, for our turn to make our point, rather than really hearing what the other person is saying. We rarely go into a conversation willing to change our views about it. We go into most situations looking to affirm our already-ingrained dogma. Many of us are afraid to upset others by speaking what is true for us, but in an advanced society I firmly believe we are all entitled to believe exactly what we want and not to be shouted down or ridiculed.

We live in a world of affirmation-seekers; we are continuously striving to reinforce the walls that we have put up in our lives that we believe protect us…but from what? Liberals watch MSNBC and conservatives watch Fox News. Both are forwarding an agenda. This is not news. This is opinion thinly disguised as news. What's the point? We will never grow if we only seek sources that reinforce our viewpoints.

But if we began each day open to learning something new, as a global society our rate of conscious expansion would skyrocket.

My beliefs are continually evolving. I will never know it all and neither will you. I certainly believe in holistic healing as I have seen it happen, and it makes sense to me and feels far less damaging to the body, but I do not shut off the valve to conventional medicine.

101

I see violence and fear all the time when people's dogmas are challenged. I used to think part of my mission was to convince people to see the world the way that I did, but now I know I am here to shine my own light. If you like it, if it illuminates your path in some way, that's great! If it doesn't, find your own truth and shine on babe.

Live each day of your life as a sponge waiting to be filled with new ideas, but ready to release it back to the river of life too. Question everything. Leave your dogma behind and observe the conflicts that you experience from another perspective. Rather than judge people who oppose your beliefs, ask them why they believe what they do. Challenge yourself to truly see the other side of the coin. If you are a Republican, get your news from MSNBC, and if you are a Democrat, give Fox News a try. Don't do this expecting to be converted, but do it instead to open yourself to understanding why those on the other side of the issue feel as strongly as they do.

We are in a time of tremendous growth and change on this planet. Change is *really* uncomfortable. It's so much easier to continue on the path that was laid for us by predecessors early on, but as Robert Frost so beautifully wrote: "Two roads diverged in a wood, and I—I took the one less traveled by, and that has made all the difference." Live your life with arms wide open, with your eyes wide open, and be prepared to be transformed. You have changed every day of your life. Change is truly the only constant, so be open to having your mind blown—it makes life far more interesting!

21.

Parenting: The Fast Track to Spiritual Enlightenment

Raising kids is part joy and part guerilla warfare.

Ed Asner

I used to look to those enlightened souls of the past and present and aspire to be like them in their grace, poise, and purity of heart. I have noticed that many of those that I admire are either women without children or whose children are raised or men who are not the primary caregiver. That is not an attainable circumstance for me, nor would I want it to be! I *love* my kids. Many wellness activists pursue their callings unhindered by the prospect of their daughter struggling with Common Core math or their son navigating the treacherous path of junior high.

Now, I recognize that those individuals leading the way to enlightenment had their own challenges to overcome, that some might have desperately wished to have children but couldn't and had to overcome that, and I certainly don't wish to diminish their experiences at all. We want to share our lives with children. We make this choice. I would never trade what I have. It does not seem reasonable or rational that God would put us all in this position if it actually stunted our spiritual growth. In fact, I now see being a primary caregiver as the AP (advanced placement) course in spiritual enlightenment.

I have often thought of writing about how to achieve spiritual enlightenment while parenting children. I always said, *When I figure it out, I'll write it.* Then I realized there was nothing to figure out. I just needed to put into practice all the lessons that I've learned. Children learn from what we do, not what we say. In fact, working with these lessons through the experience of parenting is a fast track to enlightenment. It is not for the faint of heart and is definitely not an ego massage. It is messy, unpredictable, and exhausting. Just when you think you have a win in your corner, another issue pops up that requires your undivided attention—while you simultaneously cook dinner, fold laundry, and grab the sock out of the puppy's mouth before it's torn to shreds. What do I mean by "lessons"? Here are a few examples:

Your Job Isn't to Fix Others' Problems; It Is to "Hold the Space."

Holding the space is one of those New Age phrases that basically means that you are allowing someone else to talk about their issue, to vent, to put words to it, so that they can begin to see the lesson and the solution. Holding the space is not listening to someone's problem and trying to solve it. As a parent, I know that when my kids come to me with a problem my immediate reaction is to try to solve it for them. This usually doesn't work. Occasionally I have a win, but more often my kids get frustrated by my suggestions, roll their eyes, and fail to listen to my advice. We spin our wheels.

Honestly, did your mother solve your problems growing up? I'm not talking about basic needs—I'm talking about emotional wounds. When someone was nasty to you in seventh grade, did your mom fix it? Is it reasonable to expect that a mother can fix that? Sure, you can get all *helicopter* and call the parents of all the offending kids that ever made your children feel less than, but at some point don't your children need to figure out that others' opinions should not dictate how they feel about themselves? Don't they have to go through the pain to learn how they will handle it? Didn't we all do that? Recognizing that we are not responsible for how others feel about us is a profoundly important spiritual lesson! It's a lesson I think most adults still need to learn. Instead of trying to fix the problem, the enlightened approach would be to let your child vent. Allow them to let it all out so the bad feelings don't get stuck in their bodies. Hug them. Physical touch is powerfully healing. Be quiet and be present. Send them loving energy. Remind them that you were a kid once, too, and you remember how bad it felt sometimes and that you are so sorry that they have to feel this. If it seems opportune, tell them about some of your ugly moments and share how you grew from them. Be kind and gentle and recognize that they are on a spiritual path as well. Hold the space and let them know that they can always confide in you. This isn't just kids' stuff. These are the events that shape our later experiences. Honor them.

Loving Yourself Is More Important than Anything Else You Will Ever Learn

Self-love was something I have really had to work through. I never felt that way about myself. I was far closer to the self-loathe camp. I don't know if being a kid is harder now than it was before, but it certainly carries a lot of pressure to succeed. Kids now run around from activity to activity, always proving themselves and their worth. Dance, basketball, art, swimming, debate team—although these activities lead to enrichment, they also often lead to feelings of unworthiness. It seems that kids spend a fair amount of their *free* time doing things to improve themselves. Okay, so that is the way things are now, and there is great benefit in finding what you are passionate about, but the way it's done isn't exactly a recipe for self-love, is it? When you push yourself to succeed, to be the best at something, aren't you acknowledging at some level that you wouldn't be good enough if you sucked at it? Everyone is looking for their niche, that activity that they can hang their hat on and say *I am worthy, I am good enough.* In the pursuit of spiritual enlightenment, an important step is discovering that we are all one, no one is better than anyone else, no one is more deserving. You don't need to *prove* yourself; you just need to *be* yourself. It's a bitch-slap to the ego that pretty much flies in the face of Western parenting.

I am closer to self-love than I have ever been before, but I still mess it up. I still feel as though I must prove my worth sometimes. Parenting can be like a mirror. Parenting gives us the opportunity to look at our own ego issues. It gives us the chance to demonstrate to our kids that we love ourselves even though we are far from perfect. Parenting also offers us the chance to share with our kids that trying is far more important than succeeding, even though our ego-driven world would attempt to tell them the exact opposite. Demonstrate how much you love yourself by taking excellent care of all of your physical, mental, and emotional needs. Teach your children that loving themselves for exactly who they are leads to generosity and fulfillment. Self-love is not selfish and actually makes one a better parent because it shows your child that everybody matters. Remind them (and yourself) that God made all of us. God did not make Susie more perfect or deserving than Jane.

Surrender. Let Go of Your Need to Control Your Life.

Parenting is chaos. We try so valiantly to organize, schedule, and stay on top of all that we need to do. The only friends I see around me who have this under control are people who naturally love organization and when their schedule goes awry, they go into full panic mode. You know the ones: the moms who get excited about new wall organizers. In my life at least, most of these women were teachers before having children, and thus they are in their comfort zone with managing the controlled chaos of children. For the rest of us novices, parenting provides a pretty real world lesson in surrender. Sometimes you simply can't be in three places at once. Parenting is like working the graveyard shift in a hospital emergency room on a full moon. You never know what lunacy is going to come walking through the door.

I work at home while my kids are at school. I am in total control of that environment. I decide. At 3:00 p.m., with the screech of the school bus, all bets are off. Is my daughter going to get off the bus smiling or storming into the house crying about a bad encounter with a friend? It's a crapshoot. I. Have. No. Control. I switch gears from being in control to being utterly at the mercy of the winds. My only option is to go with the flow. This is where holding the space must be put to use. Every moment in our lives offers us an opportunity to learn. As parents, we have ample opportunities to choose a different response when we screw it up the first, second, or tenth time. Sometimes I react in frustration. That does not serve my kids nor me. Instead, it behooves us all to observe the scene that we find ourselves in and respond only after mindful consideration and a deep breath (lock yourself in the bathroom for a minute if you have to). One of my favorite expressions about getting kids to do what you want is that it's like *herding cats*. So true. Life is not control. Control sucks the joy out of life and leaves no room for the unexpected. Let go. Expect the unexpected and roll with it. Surrender, and in doing so, show your kids that life is meant to be messy. The messes teach us all the most.

All That You Are Is a Result of What You Have Thought

Buddha said these wise words. I have often contemplated this spiritual truth and acknowledged that I would like to have a little chat with my higher self regarding some of the things I have created. Childhood is about distilling oneself and making choices about who you would like to be and who you wouldn't. Often the creative process is done without conscious thought, however. Practicing conscious creation, which essentially means keeping your mind on what you want to happen rather than what you don't, is an absolutely essential lesson to teach children.

You could equate it with the pessimist/optimist view of the world. Both the pessimist and the optimist achieve exactly what they put into it. The pessimist will usually be proven right that nothing works out for him. The optimist will usually be right that everything works out for the best for her. From a child's perspective, this could translate to *I'm not smart* because a standardized test failed to acknowledge that individual's unique talents, or *nobody likes me* because your child feels bad about being left out of a recess game. As we continue down our paths, we find more of these types of events because that is where our mind is being programmed to take us based on what we have previously experienced. We are master story tellers, but not always to our advantage. This is where patterns form. In these moments, we must reprogram our minds. As a parent, you need to teach your children how to change their radio station, their energetic frequency.

As parents, we are given the opportunity to lead by example in every interaction. We must model the truth that we create what we experience by appreciating when things go right and acknowledging our responsibility when things go wrong. Stop blaming others. When we blame, we are teaching scapegoating. Allow your kids to see you stating your affirmations about yourself. "I am going to make this work. I love myself. I am pretty awesome!" Allow them to see you acknowledge your snafus and course corrections, too. "Yeah, that didn't work out that well. Next time, I am going to try it this way instead. I learned a lot about what I don't want to happen." Let your kids witness your humanity, not your perfection. Teach them this power.

These are just a very small sampling of the opportunities for enlightenment that we as parents are fortunate enough to experience. Approach your challenges with humor, love, and the acknowledgement that everything that happens to us is a part of a divine plan that we created so that we could awaken fully to our true selves. In giving to our children in these ways, we also give to ourselves and get closer to remembering who we all really are.

22.

Bless It All

For everything created by God is good, and nothing is to be rejected if it is received with thanksgiving, for it is made holy by the word of God and prayer.

1 Timothy 4:4–5

Many religions and traditions teach the blessing of food before we eat it. I saw this as a lovely tradition that provided an opportunity to express gratitude, but now I realize there is more. Once I began to appreciate that our consciousness effects reality and that everything was made of energy, I began to understand that blessing something imbues it with *power.*

We are energetic beings, and everything we come in contact with has a vibration. In every instance it is wise and prudent to bless what we encounter so that it carries the highest possible vibration to support us. Recently, I have come to believe that blessing the food we eat puts an intention into it that it won't harm us and will instead strengthen us. We are experiencing a physical world, and if we move through it unconsciously, I believe the food we eat can harm or heal us depending on what we believe about it. At the highest level, however, there is no inherent good or bad until we assign a label.

It is our intention that carries the true power, but until our intention is pure, without guilt, we must obey physical laws that demonstrate fruits and vegetables to be more life supporting than Big Macs. Can I say this with scientific support? No. This is theoretical for now, but it is too thought-provoking not to share.

There was a Japanese scientist named Dr. Masaru Emoto who passed away in 2014. I was a great admirer of his work. One of his most influential experiments was with the consciousness of water. The human body is in large part water, so experimenting on the consciousness of water was also an experiment on human consciousness. I first saw this experiment in the quantum physics movie *What the Bleep do We Know!?* and was so fascinated that I read Dr. Emoto's book on his findings.

He froze water from various rivers and lakes in Japan and viewed their crystallized structures under a microscope. Some water was from pristine sources and others from polluted sources. The crystalline structures from pristine sources were beautiful and unique, reminiscent of snowflakes. The crystals from polluted water lacked cohesive form. Dr. Emoto theorized that emotional vibrations could alter the physical structure of the water. He experimented by singing to the water, attaching loving words or words of hatred to jars of water, and observing them again. No matter the source, polluted or pristine, the water that experienced love and harmonic music produced unique and beautiful crystals when frozen. The water that experienced hatred did not. It is a profound experiment and an example of consciousness affecting matter. He conducted many such experiments over several years.

I have also read so many testimonials of people who have healed their cancers naturally. From all that I have read, it is clear that there is not one diet that heals all. Some people healed with all-raw diets. Some with juicing. Some heal with cooked foods. My holistic practitioner encourages some lean animal protein, while others practice only vegan. I have read the account of a woman who took a spiritual journey after being diagnosed with cancer in which she ate predominantly corn for a few months while travelling in South America, and she healed. Corn is highly toxic for my body. People are healing with ALL of these approaches, so what's going on?

Dr. Kelly Turner identifies nine key factors that can make a real difference in healing "incurable" cancers in the *New York Times* bestseller Radical Remission: Surviving Cancer against All Odds, [5] which documents the steps taken by people who healed "incurable" cancers. While changing diet is listed as a key factor, the diets each person used were different. In fact, of the nine factors only two were physical changes—diet and natural supplements. The other seven factors were emotional and mental. The evidence continues to lead me to believe that what we think and feel is what matters most. Mind over matter!

Blessing your food, the guy that flipped you the bird on the highway, or the spider hanging out in the corner of your ceiling just makes sense in a world where your intention shapes your outcome. I realize that this is a challenging suggestion, but what do you have to lose by experimenting with it? Don't expect the Big Mac to serve you until you can, in full conscious awareness, believe that it won't hurt you. I'm not there yet, but I relish the day mint chocolate chip ice cream feeds my body and my soul!

23.

<u>Make Love, Not War</u>

Wars are poor chisels for carving out peaceful tomorrows.

Martin Luther King Jr.

How many wars are you waging right now? How many wars are you supporting? Do you support the war on drugs, cancer, inequality, or terrorism? What if war wasn't the answer?

War doesn't change the aggression and hatred in the heart. War is the perception that one side is right and the other is wrong. While I recognize that someone like Adolf Hitler had to be stopped by force, most circumstances aren't that clear cut. To be honest, had the people of Europe at the end of the First World War not tried to punish the German people so harshly through the Versailles Treaty—wreaking economic castration on Germany—Hitler would never have been in a position to rise to power. Once he did, had the people of Europe stood courageously to oppose his very first acts of aggression rather than appease him, World War II might never have happened.

Most other modern incidents of warfare have been far less noble, in my opinion. I'm sure that there have been justifications for them, but many have been flimsy and not well thought out, and some have been illusions that convinced a society to enter an ill-advised conflict to satisfy greedy agendas.

According to Albert Einstein, change cannot come from the same consciousness that created a problem. War may temporarily stop overt aggression, but the animosity will continue to fester until another opportunity presents itself for the snake of hatred to strike.

What about the war one wages when they have cancer? Cancer was something created by your own body. Why would you go to war with it? A better approach might be to finally begin to love yourself so fiercely that no room existed for anything but love. Learn to love your cancer. Thank it for the way it is changing you. It was no accident but divine design that brought it to your experience. I know that flies in the face of every cancer campaign out there, but has the war on cancer made anything better or are more people diagnosed with cancer now than at any time before?

The war on drugs has created a prison system overburdened by nonviolent drug *offenders*. The war on drugs has wasted millions of dollars and has created the backdrop for great violence in South and Central America and in our own country.

If you are at war with a person, maybe a *frenemy*, one whom you compete with passive aggressively. This person isn't your enemy. They are a child of God just like you. In fact, anything they do to piss you off is mirroring an aspect of yourself (subconsciously) that you would rather not acknowledge. I hated learning that particular lesson. I'd much rather blame someone else for making me feel bad! Alas, I know that if someone is pushing my buttons, they are helping me to see myself and clear out crap.

The next time you begin to feel the anger boiling, whether it be toward ISIS, cancer, the other side of the political aisle, or the woman in the express grocery line with well over the item limit, send them your love. Bless them, pray for them, and stay above the warped idea that war solves any problems. Love is the answer. Pretty much every spiritual teacher has told us that since the beginning of time. Ironically, I find that the most religious people also often tend to support war. Jesus was a peace activist. There is far more that unites us than divides us. Divine Love is the most powerful chemical in the universe. Will you heed the wisdom to love, a power that can heal the world, or continue to breed the destructive force of hatred?

24.

Choice Chaos

Beware the barrenness of a busy life.

Socrates

We do an excellent job of being busy. We take pride in running from task to task and event to event. It's almost a competition to stuff our weekends with activities. We buy more stuff to fill our closets. We redecorate our houses. We buy all the latest gadgets. Let's face it—consumer product companies hold immense power over us. They study us and learn how to market products that make us feel like we are missing out if we don't buy what they are selling. It's a hamster wheel of feeling good when we have a bright and shiny new object, only for the feeling to quickly fade and be replaced by the desire for the next bright and shiny object.

There seems to be a trend as we shift in consciousness away from believing that material items can bring peace and happiness. I don't believe for a second there is anything wrong with comfort. I do question the sanity of the incessant need for the new. I have been doing a lot of material purging in the last few months. I purged more than forty percent of my clothes. I see a lot of other people doing it, too.

I am at a point in my life where I want very little. I want what I have to be nice quality, but I don't need any more dishes, decorations, or clothes. I instituted a policy in which if I purchase something new, but unnecessary, *that day* I must give away two items. It makes me pause and consider whether the new sweater is worth giving away two other articles of clothing and makes me focus on whether it will really make me happier.

My friends know that I am not a fashionista. I never have been. I refuse to wear high heels unless they are truly comfortable...which usually means I don't wear heels. I normally choose to wear only my wedding ring and earrings day in and day out. Clothing is just not important enough to me to spend extra time on it. I am not label-conscious. I have the same pair of shorts from New York and Company in five different colors. I have the same turtleneck sweaters from Kohl's in five different colors. I wear comfortable jeans or leggings, boots, FitFlops, or Dansko shoes. I have two nice dresses that people see me in over and over again. There have been times when I have tried to shake things up, but I always revert to what is most comfortable for me to wear, so I am finally willing to embrace it.

I guess I'm a little like Steve Jobs on this one. I found something that I like, and I am sticking to it. By wearing the same clothes over and over again, I am freeing up my mind to focus on decisions that mean more to me. By simplifying this one thing, I made room for more of what I care about.

If you love clothes, then keep shopping and enjoying it, but find another area of your life where you overburden yourself with choices and decisions that, at the end of the day, you don't care that much about. Get to a point where you spend the majority of your time on things that matter to you and get rid of everything else you can.

Just look at TV programming options. My husband loves the choices, especially for sports. I want to turn on the TV and have HGTV, Biography, *Modern Family,* and *The Amazing Race.* Cable, for me, is choice paralysis. Most weekends when we try to choose a family movie, we get lost in the program guide for forty-five minutes! There are too many choices and too many decisions, and it sucks away my energy and my free time.

It is in the stillness of life when we make realizations that shape us, change us, and help us to grow. If you are always busy doing and focusing on minutia, you won't have time to nurture the most important relationship you have, the one with yourself.

25.

A Tumor Is like a Pearl

The world is your oyster.

William Shakespeare

By now you know that I believe whatever perspective through which we choose to view something is what we create out of any of life's experiences. At some point along my journey, I became aware of a group of scientists suggesting that a tumor is the immune system's way of saving your life. Well, if *that* didn't fly in the face of everything I had ever heard!

A tumor is not a foreign substance. It is a part of the body, created by the body. Why it's there is the subject of much debate, but consider this. If a tumor is a product of the immune system, and the immune system's job is to protect us, then maybe a tumor is an ancient mechanism of protection. With my holistic slant, because I have found it to be more on point, I believe that cancer is a state of toxicity in the body. It can be mental, emotional, and physical, and I believe it is often a combination of all three. Anita Moorjani shared in *Dying to Be Me*, her book about surviving stage IV lymphoma after a near-death experience, that she realized while on the other side of the veil that her cancer was created by her life force energy that had been suppressed for too long by fears. Her life force energy turned inward and began consuming her.

Perhaps a tumor forms to protect the body from this toxicity. Perhaps it spreads because the cause of the toxicity isn't being addressed. I know that dogs sometimes get fatty tumors at the site of vaccinations, presumably to protect the body from the vaccine additives. Why can't a tumor be a positive thing? That got me thinking about pearls and how they form.

A pearl is formed when a foreign substance—an irritant like a grain of sand—gets past the mantle of the oyster. To protect itself, the oyster begins coating the invader with layers of nacre (mother-of-pearl), which over time forms a pearl. This beautiful object is created directly from an organism's response to irritation.

The brain tumor, and any tumor for that matter, is exactly the same. My body, in its infinite wisdom, created a tumor to protect me from the toxins encased in it. Isn't that a beautiful and empowering way of appreciating the wisdom of the body? Rather than hating my body for creating a tumor, I thank it for saving me up until now.

Over time, this substance that causes the oyster stress transforms into one of the most treasured substances on earth. I have found on my journey that the brain tumor is exactly the same. It protects me at the deepest level because it encourages me to follow my soul's guidance. I wasn't embracing life before the tumor, but now I am and that is quite a gift. The brain tumor called me to change, and I heeded the call. I love my body's pearl whether it stays with me for the rest of my life or evaporates back into the ethers.

117

Onward!

I hope that the pearls of wisdom I have shared will help you to reconnect with your authentic, soul-inspired self. There is so much more to know, for me and for you. Begin to trust yourself more than you have allowed yourself before. You are wise. You are an aspect of God. Walk with that knowledge.

Live like each moment of your life is a glorious scene in a kaleidoscope—constantly changing, yet always beautiful.

Remember each day that life is eternal, but that this particular incarnation is not, so make the most of every moment.

Love,

Erin

Acknowledgments

I would like to thank my husband Mike for his unwavering support as I stopped and started the process of writing this book, working through my insecurities and ego-bullying. You are amazing. I would like to thank my children, Aidan and Kyra, for keeping me on my toes and always giving me the opportunity to keep it real while I developed my spiritual confidence. I love you both so much and am so proud of the people you are.

I would also like to thank my personal tribe of healing coaches, including Dr. Mark Mincolla, Dr. Katina Manning, Debbie McBride, Nina Koyama, Ginny May, Beth O'Connor, Nancy Thomas, Pauline Pearson, Dr. Richard Margil and Karen Paolino Correia who, in different ways and at different times, have opened my eyes to what lies beyond the veil of illusion and have enriched my life experience. Thank you so much!

References

1. Anita Moorjani, *Dying to Be Me* (California: Hay House, 2014).
2. Billy Best, *The Billy Best Story* (Massachusetts: Sandcastle Memoirs, 2012).
3. Maxwell Maltz, *The New Psycho-Cybernetics* (New Jersey: Prentice Hall, 2002).
4. Louise L. Hay, *Heal Your Body* (California: Hay House, 1984).
5. Kelley A. Turner, *Radical Remission: Surviving Cancer against All Odds* (New York: HarperCollins, 2014).

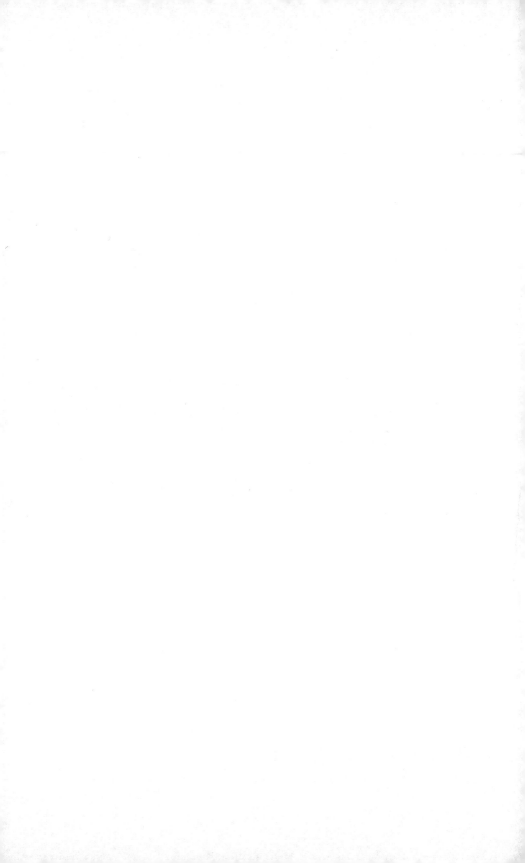

Made in the USA
Middletown, DE
01 March 2017